# MIND OVER DIET: PSYCHOLOGY, FOOD, FITNESS AND THE ART OF SELF-NEGOTIATION

Thomas S. Mueller, PhD, MBA

Copyright © 2014 ProfWriter, LLC


profwriter.com

mastercompetitor.blogspot.com

tsmueller.blogspot.com

mindoverdiet.blogspot.com

"Pain is inevitable, suffering is optional"

- Ancient Buddhist proverb

# CONTENTS

## DISCLAIMER

The ideas, concepts and opinions expressed in this publication are intended for educational purposes only. The author is not rendering medical advice of any kind or to diagnose, prescribe or treat any disease, condition, illness or injury. Before beginning any diet or exercise program, you should receive full medical clearance from a licensed physician.

The author claims no responsibility to any person or entity for any liability, loss, or damage caused or alleged to be caused directly or indirectly as a result of the use, application or interpretation of the material in this publication.

# CHAPTER ONE

## Endangered species

It would have been easy to start this book with a flattering account of my credentials regarding food, fitness and the mentality associated with successful eating habits.

However, the journey itself has not always been impressive and is pockmarked with highs and lows. It's somewhat notable that I have consistently engaged endurance sport for over 30 years. I have finished dozens of triathlons, over 50 marathons and just as many ultramarathon runs, including eight (8) 100-mile finishes. That accomplishment is something to relish and also ponder. My life is viewed through the lens of the long, slow journey and on a good day, an eventual finish.

What a wild ride it has been. I have struggled through hypothermia on my bicycle, went into anaphylactic shock from a bee sting, suffered heat exhaustion on a dusty road 85 miles into ultrarunning race and waited out lightning strikes in a cave atop a mountain in West Virginia.

My quest towards healthy living began in 1983. I was in a fast-paced PR job that entailed traveling to sport and entertainment events across the USA. It was time to face the fact I ate too much, consumed too much alcohol, didn't exercise, and carried a hefty 214 pounds on a portly frame.

The passion came into me. I power-dieted and lost 45 pounds that fall, living on peanut butter sandwiches, frozen low calorie dinners and baked potatoes. My weight eventually plateaued at 165 pounds and set a new standard. A "set point" had been calibrated.

I incorporated running and cycling, until I was capable of completing my first "biathlon" (running and cycling) the following spring. That led to several seasons of triathlon racing, then my first marathon in 1987. A year later the ultramarathon bug bit me and I completed the Mountain Masochist 50-mile run in Virginia.

Nothing remains more elusive, and ultimately epic, than a 100-mile ultramarathon finish. It's that point in time when your body screams stop, again and again, hour after hour. Yet you tell your brain that you can do it, that you're good enough and that it's worth it in the end. You finish the race, earn a fleeting validation, and move forward.

There's actually more to it than that. Maybe it's my arsenal of running shirts that I wear with jeans, or my warmed over running shoes that serve as daily footwear. Or it may come down to the strength that has built inside, the power that guides me when career and relationship pressures weigh heavy on my shoulders. I apply my running acumen to the challenge; circumstances may hurt but I will complete the task.

There's another dimension, outside of endurance sport, which has defined my being. This is the 20th anniversary of my victory over Guillain-Barre Syndrome. GBS is an autoimmune dysfunction. Somehow, my body read the wrong signals from a flu shot and started to eat the myelin sheaths from around my nerves. When the nerves misfired my body short circuited. Soon, I was a living being inside a shell that did not move or breathe.

The descent into GBS came quickly. It was November 1992; I can remember the election count coming in as Bill Clinton shifted into the lead. My vision started to fuzz out, my arms stopped working and then my legs stopped supporting my weight.

At first, I languished in a local hospital while a general practitioner tried to kill me (my opinion). I was transferred to a regional hospital in an ambulance, but on the way my attending nurse barfed all over the floor due to motion sickness. This might have been funny, if I wasn't in the process of dying as my lungs shut down.

I did make it to the regional hospital, which is a good thing, as it allows me to tell you this story. I called the intensive care unit home for the next 11 days, slipping in and out of morphine doses and a completely paralyzed state. Each breath was a little puff of oxygen coming in and out of the respirator. A knowledgeable neurologist saved my life by administering 13 plasmapheresis treatments. Think of plasmapheresis as an oil change for the body. The process extracts all of one's blood and filters the albumen. These treatments made me stronger each session.

During my early stages of recovery in January, 1994, I mentioned to a nurse that I wanted to complete the Ice Age Trail 50-mile run that May. She chuckled and said, "You'll be lucky to be shuffling down the hallway in a walker."

My point is this: The nurse underestimated my ability and conviction, just as many will underestimate your will to succeed as you work through your Mind over Diet rejuvenation plan. I finished Ice Age that year. The key to success was a slow, methodical effort over a long period of time. I used my heart rate monitor as a tool and never let my pulse rise higher than 130 beats per minute. I conserved energy and clawed my way to the finish.

Knock me down, I'll get back up. Tell me I'll be shuffling in a walker, and I'll show you how I run.

But that was then and this is now. There is no need to thrive on the past, unless it benefits the future. What I have learned is that we'll never know when our time on this earth is about to end and it's time to head for the exit door. My GBS experience set a benchmark going forward. I am enjoying bonus time and with the days that remain, I want to live well and help others.

Though I might have shattered some physical barriers, a negative dimension weaved its way into my athletics and health issues. It was the pseudo victories and sometimes painful defeats related to eating and nutrition. For several decades, I was self-defined by endurance sport, rather than nutrition and health. I used race finishes to compensate for other less rewarding dimensions of my life.

Relationship issues, financial matters and work stress many times trigger bad behavior. My weight crept up in five-pound increments, on some occasions cresting the 180-pound mark. Then I'd get mad, set my ultramarathon mindset into motion, and eliminate the errant pounds. I would tolerate the distasteful (literally) weight loss process until I could declare victory when weight "X" was achieved. Sound familiar? Can you relate to those days, peering down past your toes at the number calibrated on your scale?

After time, the fat gravitated back to my belly, so I started yet another comeback plan. I was motivated by a "get skinny and go fast" training routine. I lost 16 pounds over the next couple of months, overcame food binge setbacks, and felt light and fit.

The results took me to a place unknown since high school—155 pounds. But the price to get there was high. I had to filter the accomplishment through the ravaged body of a 50-something athlete. There's some sort of weight vs. fitness vs. aging formula I have yet to invent.

When it comes to losing weight, my closest friend, and subsequent adversary, is running. I come back to that dangerous mistress time and again, embracing her on 10-mile outings every morning.

*Thin is in, fat is not where it's at…thin is in, fat is not where it's at.* I'd chant that mantra as I ran, spurring my pace as the miles slipped by. In my world, I was flying. My pace dropped under nine minutes per mile and a warm breeze caressed my face. My breath wasn't labored and I wasn't fighting the climbs. My stride lengthened as I flowed down the next descent.

I loved the exhilaration that came with increased fitness, but it always came back to heartbreak when physical degeneration toppled me back to reality. The running would subside and I'd slip back into bad eating habits. I might sustain a good level of training, but I'd eat my way past that effort. As my weight increased, my attitude once again slipped into a gloomy place.

Over this past summer, the vicious cycle continued. I gained 20 pounds and 5% body fat. I was satiating my immediate desires but stifling my long term well-being. My nutrition and fitness program was a house built on sand foundation. My mental state propagated a less than satisfactory end result. There was little preparation in sustaining what must be accomplished after the goal is attained.

Then, I found a better way. This book is about that journey and a path to long term success. For you see, sustaining the sweet spot begins, and ends, in the mind.

I set aside decades of head knowledge from reading and research and instead became an experiment of one. One body, one mind, and one explicit end goal: A consistent, manageable life plan that will sustain my physical and psychological well-being over years to come.

Three months later, the Mind over Diet philosophy has brought me to a 21 pound weight loss. I'm magazine cover lean at 3% body fat, enjoying my exercise, and am engaging a positive and productive attitude that I have not known since I was in my teens.

Mind over Diet is different from many other books on the market. I won't recommend any specific products, brands or parameters. I'll explain various mental, emotional and physical tasks and will be asking you to engage in "homework" that will assist in building ownership of your own personal Mind over Diet nutrition and fitness plan. Each task will be set in bold face type, so watch for those indications as you read.

The steps in this book will require research, most all of which can be conducted with a computer that accesses the Internet. I'd suggest you use your favorite search engine to identify content related to the task I suggest. As an author, I want to be inclusive of all readers. If you aren't active on computers, or possibly don't have Internet connection access, consider visiting your local library, and then speak with the reference librarian. I'm sure most will be happy to assist in your study.

Mind over Diet won't try to sell you specific plans or timelines. It won't promise an intended result. Rather, we'll take this journey together and work to restructure your psychological foundation, just as I did through my own rebirth. This is a process that you'll engage on your own terms, with deliverables that you will design and approve. With authorship comes pride of ownership. No one will tell you how to succeed; you'll be designing that road map as you accomplish step-by-step tasks and gain knowledge. A trainer won't be standing over you, demanding the next stomach crunch or dead lift. Instead, you'll self-negotiate your food intake, exercise and tracking mechanisms.

I hope you'll enjoy this expedition towards a new beginning as much as I did. You're an experiment of one, and the new journey is underway. This is the day you begin a Mind over Diet transformation in your life.

# CHAPTER 2
## Psychology

We've all embraced (or succumbed to) to the following private moment. It's after a shower or when donning apparel for the day to come. You turn, face a full length mirror and stare.

It's the naked test.

Who do you see? What emotions and responses does the person in the mirror evoke? Are you at peace with the image in front of you, or disgusted with what you see?

What the naked test teaches is that we really can't hide from ourselves and our perceptions. If the outcome is good, or bad, we must face the person who stares back at us and determine what took us to our current point in life.

Much of our reaction to the naked test is generated by the pattern of thought within our minds. We preconceive ourselves and the world around us. We organize and process incoming information and add it to our "schema"−our cognitive (fact based) framing mechanism that helps us order and interpret the world around us. Many times, a negative schema can support and enforce the wrong messages. Schemas order our thoughts and operate in the background, helping us make sense of daily outcomes. Stereotypes, perceived social roles, and our overall worldviews are affected through perceptions of schema.

Schemas represent a collection of thoughts in our brains. It's how we assemble facts and experiences over time, to determine what is "right" and how things work within our lives. Many times, our schemas engage on a subconscious level, helping us to process incoming information.

Our minds tend to accept and embrace thoughts and events that coincide with our schema; if we are part of an occurrence that conflicts with schema, we enter a period of cognitive dissonance – that of trying to find a point of agreement between our schema and this new information. We may bump up against contradicting beliefs and experience mental stressors that make us uncomfortable.

There's a substantial amount of cognitive dissonance within the multi-billion dollar diet and weight loss industry. We may have built a schema over several years, embracing the mandate that if you want to run well, and run far, eat carbs the night before a race. A big spaghetti dinner with whole grain bread may be the proposed best meal.

Then, advocates of the Paleo Diet suggest that most carbs are bad, protein and good fats are primary sources, and that grains are out of bounds. Our cognitive dissonance rages as we sort out what we thought we believed and what we now intend to adopt.

There are other messy parts in your schema, disassociated facts that have clumped together to form unintended outcomes. For example, you may have validated eating as a numbing agent for psychological pain, boredom or depression. Your schema may be direct-wired to command "food!" whenever stress crosses your path. Or your schema may have tracked past experience and convinced your psyche that food is equated to failure and your inability to be successful in attaining and sustaining good eating habits and a toned body.

On some occasions our schemas can promote a less than productive outcome. When we have unmet needs and feel lonely, stressed, or angry, we may produce clustered reasoning that states food or possibly alcohol can satiate the unstable state of mind. Of course, there can be both psychological and physical motivators in play, but surely our mind takes the lead in justifying food as numbing agent.

When false perceptions become the norm, another significant dimension in your diet and fitness journey comes into play. Social identity is your self-concept of "membership" in a perceived social group. Some social identities are detrimental, such as "I am overweight" or "there is no way I can run."

Other indicators of social identity are captured in the graphics featured on apparel. You may be proud to carry the colors and logo of your favorite sport team or you may choose to visually associate with the name and logo of a university or college. Demonstrating our "club" is many times tied to our perceived social worth.

For example, social identity with sedentary groups can impair one's motivation to succeed in diet and fitness. I have no issue with being a fan of collegiate or professional football, but the activities surrounding football games might include an abundance of food, subsequent overindulgence, and enforcement of the "live to eat" mentality.

Social identities with outdoor lifestyle groups, walking clubs or recreational sport teams can motivate our behavior, build a health-related schema and reduce bouts with negative outcomes.

Your social identity may have been hijacked. Downsizing at work might have turned you into a 65-hour-a-week company drone. This isn't the true internal you, but rather a fractured version that has been propagated through fear, job instability and expectations in a competitive marketplace.

On other occasions, social identity can slip into your role within family functions, leadership at civic organizations, or the "go to" as a friend or companion. There is nothing wrong with any of these activities, but when your self-perception identifies any of these identities as essential, you may have lost the balance necessary for personal wellness and active living.

I will interject that during a period of my life endurance sport activities defined my social identity. Looking back, it all became rather crazy. I built a shrine in my basement workout area, with posters of myself competing in mountain bike and ultradistance races. Medals and race number bibs were framed and mounted for display.

When troubles came in the form of relational distress and business failures, I became desperate to maintain the ultradistance racer facade. There were 100-mile races where my social identity was so skewed I told myself I had to finish in order to validate and sustain my ultrarunning status; all else in life looked bleak. Being aware of how you perceive yourself is paramount in creating a sustainable Mind over Diet outcome.

Another psychological element that affects how you approach your engagement with diet and fitness is a predisposition to either introvert or extrovert behavior. There are large populations of introverts who don't sync well with the show and tell version of body transformation. On many occasions introverts play out as a disadvantaged segment of society. They may not be outgoing and can experience heightened stress levels through forced interaction.

For an introvert, there is a real, tangible fear associated with unwanted attention. Introverts may recharge through reading, thought and introspection. The rewards of life may be found in quieter places, not through "look at me" imaging of ripped torsos and muscled arms.

Extroverts may become supercharged through their fitness and nutrition experience. As body fat decreases and muscle increases, extrovert consumers may gain motivation through complements, comments and other interactions.

However, if extroverts suffer a setback, they may drop out of site and away from the Mind over Diet plan for success. This is a common outcome in recreational competition; when extroverts stop winning age group awards, they many times exit the sport. Without the public recognition of winning, they disconnect from the food, exercise and competition that fed the related recognition.

Psychological filters such as introversion or extroversion, schemas and social identity can affect our ability to be lean, strong and happy. We may not realize that our minds have become preset through years of negative input, bad advice or relational struggles. Some may have suggested you look better "with a few extra pounds on your bones" or that "you're getting too thin, you don't look healthy." Or, at family gatherings or dinners out, you might hear "it's a special occasion" as your plate is filled a second time, or "the bread pudding here is a must." Please understand I am not stating that indulging on special occasions is wrong, but I will suggest that when your behavior is affected by the messaging of others, it's reason to beware.

You might have repetitive failures at losing weight. Maybe your schema suggests you are destined to be "fat." It's possible your social identity is tied to being the grill master of your neighborhood, which in turn leads to over eating and invariably back to standing in front of the mirror, naked, with a gloomy vision of the future. Or, your introverted nature has been a barrier to the local fitness facility, as the close proximity of people is just too much to tolerate.

At many points in my life, individuals and social groups have prompted me to exit into the shadows. I was told I was too untalented, or too slow, or too unrealistic for my intended outcome. It's as if others who have succumbed to a paunchy caricature of themselves wanted me to join their social identity group. Overtures are made to gain a few pounds and exercise less. Running is bad for your knees anyway, correct? Why push it at your age? They'd suggest it would be better if I gave up and blended into the landscape.

In order combat these negative inputs, I hold an allegorical vision in my mind. It is of a football field during a night game, engulfed in bright, encompassing light. But just beyond the boundaries of the field, the sidelines are murky and dark. Both internal and external forces in my life have told me to stay on the sidelines of life, to remain in the shadows. These forces want to push me away from success, to accept less than optimum as good enough.

Deep inside of us all is the will, the power, the exceptional nature to succeed. It can manifest itself in a deep and reverent way, intrapersonal in nature. We can run into the open and scream "No more sidelines for me, I'm running into the light, I'm running onto the field! I want to get into the game!"

As with all things in Mind over Diet, I'm not advocating that one's psychological disposition is in any way a handicap. There are no perfect psychological profiles and there's no perfect path to the healthy, fit individual you will become. What is important is that you acknowledge who you are and which psychological motivators guide your perceptions and behavior.

No one can force you to make a psychological change. But someone can show you the path to learn and ponder and grow. Sometime during your Mind over Diet experience, you will come upon a period of cognitive dissonance. In simplest form, this is the event where you face mental discomfort, attempting to rectify what you believed to be true with a new, incongruent belief that has recently surfaced. Your brain's hard drive is trying to reboot and you're trying to facilitate and come to terms with the process.

Maybe it's the dissonance of "my family doesn't exercise and neither do I" as conflicted with "I like to run and it's time to upgrade my athletic apparel." Or, "I've always been overweight" versus "I'm going to opt out of that pot luck tonight because what I really want is a protein and green plant smoothie." What was once the norm, no longer exists. Schemas shift, social identities alter, and new lives are underway.

That's the journey we'll be on throughout this book. We'll unpack and explore the essential components of building a sustainable diet and fitness plan. You adapt along the way. Your schema can shift and your social identity can move from sport watching to sport participation.

You may become enlightened and learn that an introverted personality can be supported and nourished through the Mind over Diet protocol. Or, if you're extroverted, you may wish to engage others and challenge them to join you in developing their own Mind over Diet personal life plan.

Picture your mind as a hard drive in a computer and your psychological profile as files in that hard drive. We create files, drag them into folders, and then rank the folders into a preferable order. When you engage the Mind over Diet process you'll be creating new content, bringing some well needed documents into that mix, and shifting pertinent data into easy access. It's a RAM function in your brain!

Awareness of your personal psychological makeup is essential. Some might suggest the world around us affects our behavior, but I would suggest that how we process the world around us holds the major opportunities for improvement. When you understand more deeply than before, you have attained knowledge. Knowledge is power. Power leads to change. And change leads to success.

*Chapter Summary*

- Self-perception is either a motivator, or detractor, in your personal quest.

- Our mind orders life events and lessons; it compartmentalizes the information and creates a schema that directs how we perceive the world.

- Food holds a special place in our schemas; it represents many uses and eventual outcomes.

- When our schema comes into conflict with external messaging, we encounter cognitive dissonance and experience mental stress and discomfort.

- We strive to become associated with select groups and factions of people. Our social identity drives our motivations and actions.

- We engage an introvert, or extrovert, personality. How we interact in society is directed by personality type.

- We utilize psychological filters to make sense of our lives.

- There is an opportunity to reorder our schemas and build alternative perspectives and motivators.

- An altered schema can help alleviate cognitive dissonance and shift our perceptions to a positive, healthy social identity.

# CHAPTER 3
## Tools for success

When I teach advertising courses, it's important to help students differentiate "push" and "pull" messaging. Push messages shout the content at consumers, hoping to influence purchasing decisions. Pull messaging is permission based; it's a scenario where marketers ask consumers if they can start a conversation, hoping that potential customers will take the initiative to engage.

I want to use "pull" messaging in my approach to Mind over Diet. I want your permission to introduce a new paradigm for health and nutrition. I'll offer suggestions, give examples, and set parameters that will help you make a personal decision to engage the process.

I'm writing to you from a new round of fitness engagement. The path is never perfect, but I have been able to climb another peak in personal fitness (of course, that's an age and injury corrected assessment). I'm six feet, 1 inch tall, carrying 154 pounds on a now lanky frame. The new psychologically sound plan has allowed me to lose 22 pounds and 5% body fat over a 10-week period. My muscles are defined in an endurance sport fashion. The emotional and mental residuals are huge. Each day is a new opportunity and fears have subsided.

And for the first time in a long time, it's not a struggle. I'm comfortable with my diet and am actually working to *increase* calorie intake, to build muscle mass and maintain my target weight. I'm not hungry, don't have food on the brain 24/7 and have an overwhelming feeling of success throughout each day.

My recent success is the impetus to write Mind over Diet. This book is about struggle with food choices, about good intentions that faded over the course of time. It's about failed attempts at moderation, relapses and binges, and the dark cloud that follows when the road back seems insurmountable.

There are hundreds of diet and weight loss books available for purchase, much of it driven by the $60 billion diet industry. There are 100 million dieters looking for solutions. It's possible you have digested (pun intended) many of them. Some will suggest you live on grapefruit, while others might recommend you forage for nuts and leaves as did our Paleolithic ancestors. You may have labored with best intentions, but the outcome you achieved was inadequate and unsuccessful.

I'm not going to spoon-feed you advice on food or exercise or supplements. It's my opinion that you don't need additional challenges to achieve eating and workout advice. I'm not here to sell you anything (accept this book!) but rather want you to take ownership, to take the next step, and negotiate (with yourself) the best possible diet and fitness plan.

You are an experiment of one. I want to propose that by employing the Mind over Diet development plan, you will devise a solution that works. Mind over Diet can assist in building the plan you can sustain, indefinitely, no end game. I'll identify incremental steps that will assist you in how to access, absorb and take ownership of the necessary information.

With the tools in place, it's possible to assemble a diet and fitness plan that you personally develop and own. Success won't come from being told what to do, but in setting your own strategies and eventual outcomes. When you create it, you own it. The decisions are yours. If you choose to authorize a change in your current plan, there's only one individual who holds the authority to modify the outcome. That person is you.

Mind over Diet is an alternative to what you have attempted in the past. It's a simple to understand, logical approach that isn't mired in calculations or scientific jargon. It won't promise a 20 pound weight loss in six weeks, or fat-free washboard abs. Rather, this is a new start that will help you reframe your perceptions and better manage your daily food and fitness experience. Once these new realities of consumption are in place, you'll be able to embrace your diet plan, build self-confidence, enjoy an improved outlook and attitude, and develop a life-long wellness routine that you will personally design.

Many diet and fitness consumers take the route of a personal trainer or coach. Please understand I am not against this form of encouragement and direction, but I don't believe it's the best path to longevity and a sustained approach. Most trainer plans are driven by a near-term outcome (lose a certain amount of weight, run a faster half marathon, attain the elusive "washboard abs"). A trainer or coach can take you to that end result, but most all of that journey will entail a prescriptive "push" approach – do this, eat that, accomplish a certain goal by a certain date.

I recently heard a podcast where a well-known trainer stated that many of his clients fall off the plan, once they move beyond the coaching. Many who achieve results derived in that fashion might attain rather immediate success, but without the trainer and the input and the daily instruction, it's not going to continue over an extended period of time.

That's what is different about Mind over Diet. It's a guided tour into your own psyche, leading to personal, emotional and physical enhancements. There are no shortcuts or magic formulas; change must start from the inside and cannot be imposed. This is your opportunity to set the mental foundation needed to design an effective plan that works for you.

Gaining a new awareness, one that is empowered to succeed, will help you manage each day and note positive results. Food and fitness is no longer the enemy. A number on the scale is no longer the goal.

Feeling comfortable and relaxed in your food consumption habits isn't only possible, it's probable. Mind over Diet will help you build the "tool kit" needed to succeed.

There's an appropriate analogy in approaching the tasks to come. Consider it a morning walk through your neighborhood, where the sun has just peaked above the tree line. The air is fresh and you hold a methodical, relaxed pace. Left foot, right foot, left foot, right foot…each step intentional, yet relaxed and enjoyable. That's our journey through Mind over Diet.

The program will make you an informed, directed individual who knows what factors will bring a satisfying outcome. You are a thinking, athletic machine. Soon, you will know what high performance food you'll choose to eat and what body-enhancing activities you'll opt to engage. It won't be hard, it won't be impossible, because the plan is 100% owned by you. No one will be promising short cuts or easy fixes. This is your time, your season to become exactly what you set out to be.

Let's take a few steps forward, and begin.

*Chapter summary*

- "Pull" marketing asks for your permission; Mind over Diet is a guided tour that asks your permission to help you set new diet and fitness initiatives.

- There are hundreds of diet plans and millions of dieters. This book does not adhere to any specific plan or process. You create the plan and process.

- When you research and plan it, you own it. Ownership is powerful and builds the psychology needed to succeed.

- Many coaches and trainers push for near-term outcomes. Mind over Diet is designed to adapt your psyche for personal, emotional and physical well-being over your life span.


- Your new awareness will take you through a daily walk that is methodical, relaxing and enjoyable. It's not about immediate results; it's about the long term journey.

# CHAPTER 4

## Measuring progress

What should I eat? When should you eat it? How much is an acceptable amount? Should I ingest supplements? What is the latest diet plan? What's the fastest way to lose weight?

There is a primary universal rule regarding human beings and food: Some people eat to live. Other people live to eat.

I was recently visiting a friend. This individual is in his late 50's, rail thin, and is an accomplished bicyclist. His wife brought in two large pizzas and of course, the accompanying cooked dough sticks that melt in your mouth.

My athletic friend ate 1.5 pieces of pizza and pushed all the boxes aside. This individual represents the "eat to live" model. Food is fuel, sustenance that the body needs to perform. It's easy for eat to live humans to be around all sorts of food because their foundational psychology allows it. Food has its place and holds no other diabolical attraction.

Then, there are the rest of us. We "live to eat" and use food for enjoyment, as a numbing drug, and to avoid the pangs of stress, depression or other emotions. Food becomes a deterrent to a clear outlook on life. Food will satiate your senses and also increase the distance around your belt line. Food preoccupies spaces in our mind, it creates opportunities for failure, and in the worst scenarios food becomes our god.

The psychology of "live to eat" can come upon us in waves. We suppress this mental function for a while, but then it once again roars into our lives. Unlike my bicyclist friend, I can't view that plethora of pizza as anything less than a mass of delicious treasure, waiting to be conquered. There's no 1.5 pieces for me; rather it's one (pizza) until done.

Based on obesity statistics for the United States – and now many other regions of the world – it's safe to note that we no longer control our food choices. Rather, food controls us.

Attempting to negotiate through today's maze of diet and nutrition information is a relentless challenge. We can explore books, watch TV shows, follow a never-ending array of Internet and social media sources, listen to a podcast, or rely to word of mouth from others who are also on the weight loss quest.

My motivation to publish this book was incubated when I began working on my food intake in a methodical fashion over a three month period. I'm a social scientist, so I began by engaging a research model: Compile existing information, determine how to assimilate data, categorize intended food content into heterogeneous groupings, benchmark food intake at start of the experiment, modify to intended food intake, and then quantify results.

During my testing months, I was in position to focus on my nutrition plan with few distractions and also exercise consistently; we'll discuss these other variables in future chapters. The outcome was exceptional. I eliminated unneeded pounds and reduced body fat. It's important to note that during this revised Mind over Diet process, I retained muscle. I brought my weight down but did my best to protect my muscle mass.

During prior weight loss efforts, I thought light would make me a faster runner, but instead light meant cannibalizing my muscles and growing weak and frail. As we age, we need to be strong and agile, not frail and inflexible. On the nutrition front, that means filling our engines with muscle-promoting fuel.

Weight loss can also present the unintended consequence of limiting strength. I was light but sluggish and didn't have the "snap" that's needed to be happy and successful as we navigate each day.

**Your first task is to explore and choose a web source or smart phone app that calculates calories ingested, then burned through food intake and exercise.**

We'll get started by learning about how to capture what we eat, what's in what we eat, and also the expenditures we produce through exercise. There are numerous options available on the Internet, some accessed through web links and others available as applications for smart phones. I'd consider exploring through your favorite search engine; try "calorie counter" or "fitness apps" to access a targeted list of potential tools that will help you start your Mind over Diet journey.

Many of the online programs or smart phone apps are free of charge. Please examine several of the top ranked options for ease of use, visual layout and daily summary profiles, and the option to input both food and exercise components.

I'd suggest you look for a food calculator that accesses a large database of food products – when you type in your item, it will automatically bring up the brand or food group for easy capture and insertion into your daily log. The online tool that I utilize recently went through a substantial upgrade and now delivers a wide array of reports for summarizes my food intake for each day. I can proportionally track carbs, fats and protein within the food groups I have ingested, as well as other pertinent dimensions such as sodium, calcium or sugars.

Your diet and fitness tool should also integrate with fitness activities. Choose an option that can approximate and log the calories expended for various forms of exercise over inputted segments of time. For example, you make take a walk for 30 minutes. If I input "walking" my app gives various approximate paces and I choose "brisk." The app then inputs 203 calories earned for that effort.

We'll be charting all forms of activity beyond sedentary living. There is a calorie expenditure when we walk, jog, stretch, cycle, lift heavy things, pedal a bike or splash in the water. All of it is part of our Mind over Diet calculation and all of it will become measured.

When I engage my fitness and nutrition program, the favorite daily statistics are overall calories burned (through exercise) and a summary report (reported in grams) within a pie chart that illustrates total proportional intake of protein, fat and carbs for that day.

I could simply promote my tool of choice, but that's inconsistent with the Mind over Diet process. Here's where you begin to build your knowledge base, learn and understand more about what's available, and about how specific tools will serve your needs. You will assess the pros and cons of various diet and fitness tools, and then choose the option that works for you. Please understand that your input and measurement tool is highly personal, in that you will be interacting with it every day.

Most of you will choose a computer based option, but a few of you may wish to go old-school and calculate on your own. If this is your wish, consider buying one of many readily available books that documents food products and related calories content as well as protein, carbs, fat, sodium, etc. You'll also need a legal pad or notebook and a calculator.

**Now it's time to determine how many calories you ingest each day.**

You're on assignment for the next seven days. Some aspects of this process may seem tedious and at times unpleasant. You will build more files for your psychological schema, in this instance logging your normal food patterns and content. We'll look for averages and trends across a one week period.

Please understand this is not a perfect, or always specific, process. Set up the nutrition program you chose, make sure you have a user log-in, and then input whatever goes into your mouth. Some of you will have full-time access to your computer or smart phone, while others will need to jot down your food items for later entry.

Most of the online nutrition programs have user memories; when you enter certain food items multiple times, it will retain them and recall that item when you type the first few characters. What I have found is that when one is eating unencumbered, the food data entry can become daunting. If you aren't sure about a certain food, or are unsure of the quantity – guess. For example, you may have baked beans on your plate, but knowing the specific type, or amount, may be difficult. Make your best approximation and enter the item.

Stay mentally aware of all forms of food. That includes juice, regular soft drinks, alcoholic drinks and half and half in coffee. It all adds up and it all needs to be entered in your diet tracker. You may encounter cognitive dissonance when you tally food and note total calories, versus what prior perception might have indicated. Despite this mental discomfort, embrace it, lean in, and keep entering the data.

Self-education is essential as you benchmark where you are and where you intend to go.

After a week of data has been collected, play with it. What are your calorie totals for each day? Were some days exceptionally higher than others? Were most of the days tallied similar in calorie count? What is the average number of calories consumed (for this calculation, simply add the calorie totals over the seven days, and then divide by 7).

Whatever your numbers represent, they are good numbers for your purposes. You now have awareness of how many calories are ingested on a non-managed eating regimen. Rest in who you are and where the journey begins. Knowledge is power and you have just become empowered through the initial steps in Mind over Diet process.

**Your next step is to research how many calories are recommended per day for your age, height and activity levels.**

Head back to your favorite Internet search engine and enter "calories per day." This will get you started down a path of exploration. You'll come upon several calorie calculators for weight loss; remember that the key assignment is to determine how many calories are needed per day, in a sedentary state. I like to consider this as a day where I don't exercise, go to work (at my desk) and eat. What amount of calories will keep me weight-neutral on that given day?

Different sources may suggest different calorie intakes. Here's another instance where Mind over Diet takes an alternative approach. I'm not going to weigh in (pun intended!) and help you make these important decisions. As a living, thinking creature, it's up to you to sift the information provided. What makes the most sense, and why? Decision-making is another important step in owning your custom plan and adhering to it.

Another beneficial aspect of this process goes beyond the task at hand. You'll be self-educating as you read, collecting facts on weight loss, calories expended, variances in sedentary versus active lifestyles, and recommendations from fitness and medical professionals. It's schema building at its finest and it's also a social identity shifting activity. It's no longer simply about who or what you affiliate with and what you were told. You can look back on the calorie charting exercise, now explore preferred calorie intake recommendations, and then connect the dots. It's your life, it's your plan and you are building the foundation to succeed!

After study and consideration, set a calorie intake per day that makes sense for you. Have you considered several sources, and the variables they addressed in assessing the recommended caloric burn? Please ponder this step carefully, as the number you choose will be foundational in charting progress.

So, what's the gap between your actual food consumption and the intended daily caloric intake? Is there a big gap between the two, or are you overeating or possibly under eating? There's no right or wrong, just the facts and our need to build the Mind over Diet plan around the numbers. Many times a "good" day will end with the base calories under control, while at other times you may be traveling or on holiday and the calorie count can double (two days calories in one?).

A day out of range does not constitute failure. Simply dial back into a feasible eating style (I'm writing this just before meeting a friend and former teacher for a fine Mexican dinner). Life can't consistently be regimented, but we do need to know where we have been, where we are going, and when we veer off the intended path.

**Research and then determine how many calories burned equate to one pound of fat loss.**

There's no perfect science to benchmarking, then measuring your caloric intake. But as a general rule, it's a psychological advantage to gauge days that are over the "norm" on calories and those days where your Mind over Diet plan creates a deficit. I do like to acknowledge the magic number associated with a pound of blubber.

On some occasions, I have notched exceptional days where I ran 10 miles in the morning, then jammed out a 2-3 hour high intensity mountain cycling ride in the evening. Couple that with a moderate day of eating and it's possible to leave a pound somewhere on the roads just traveled. There are successes and failures, but I can assure you that on those occasions when the burn is greater than the food ingested, you will embrace the accomplishment and drop some positive bytes into your schema files.

You may find different approximations that relate a pound of fast loss. That's another piece of Mind over Diet engagement that I find exciting, in that the knowledge base shifts and we strive to stay informed.

We have covered a substantial amount of information. We have tracked calories, assessed what our daily calorie limit should be, and came upon an approximation for what it takes to lose a pound of fat. Now, we'll take steps necessary to identify a piece of equipment that's essential for your Mind over Diet program.

**Research, then purchase a scale that measures weight and body fat composition.**

A good search term to plug into your favorite Internet search engine is "fitness scales." There is a wide array of products, some in simpler form, while others go all the way with body metrics such as weight, body fat, and body mass index. Some of the top products offer wireless sync options with sport watches or fitness bracelets. There are many price points, so find a product that fits your budget. I have a pound and body fat scale that I bought about 15 years ago and it continues to serve me well. For the purposes of our Mind over Diet plan, a basic scale that provides weight and body fat will be sufficient.

All scales won't be calibrated to exacting, similar readings. Ever thought you weighed a certain weight, then got on the doctor's scale and it read something quite different? Most important is that you use the same scale every time you chart your stats. A scale will be consistent with itself, so you'll have proper feedback from inception of your program throughout the course of time.

I have scraps of paper around my office that have weight and body fat readings from more than a decade.

Some of my note taking wasn't fancy, but I marked down date, weight and body fat each time I measured. That sort of information reads like a diary and it's something you will treasure in the years to come.

Working with a scale is a two-edged sword. It can act as both friend and enemy. But let's be clear, a scale is a tool, rather than an idol to be worshiped or served. Use your scale in moderation, on a rather inconsistent basis, to chart progress and simply to recognize intermittent progress points.

Since the Mind over Diet plan doesn't have an end-point, we don't set goal weights. Programs that promise a certain amount of weight loss create a race-to-the-finish mentality. Mind over Diet proponents develop their plan, execute it, then adapt and modify as needed. The scale provides a measuring stick.

Are you ready to forge ahead? There are many elements in this journey and you are now deep into the essentials in your amazing transformation. We'll talk more about personal expectations when we delve into nutrition planning.

*Chapter summary*

- Research popular computer and/or smart phone apps that track diet and fitness. Choose one and install it.

- With your app in place, enter everything you eat over a one week period. Benchmark your current caloric intake.

- Research several sources and determine a goal caloric intake for each day.

- Research and determine how many approximate calories burned represent one pound of fat loss.

- Research, then purchase a scale that tracks weight and body fat percentage.

# CHAPTER 5

## Nutrition

Your groundwork is complete. It's time to put the gears in motion and begin your Mind over Diet transformation.

Look back at your 7-day food summaries. Observe the totals on each day for carbohydrates, protein and fats (these will be represented as grams). Do you see trends in your data? Do you see a proportion between the three, that is, what percent of 100 do carbs, fats and proteins represent?

These three categories, more than any other, will provide your Mind over Diet measuring stick. We'll learn more about which foods contribute the key content that will build your body and fuel the engine with clean burning product.

Here's a key initiative in the Mind over Diet progression: When you source and target the proper proportions of carbs, proteins and fats, your body composition will change. We have already determined how many calories you plan to ingest each day. Now, we will decide how to manipulate the food content within those calorie parameters.

Let's take our first steps into the creation of your custom Mind over Diet nutrition plan:

**Research the "experts" and explore the proposed amounts of protein per day, expressed as grams of protein per pound of body weight.**

Note the various sources you encounter on the Internet. You will see a wide range of proposed protein intakes. Look carefully; what are the underlying motivations of these sources? For example, a vegan site may have a particular position on how much protein is necessary, while a protein supplement manufacturer may have an alternative opinion. As in all things Mind over Diet, you are in command. Read, ponder and consider how you will test each source and then apply it to your personal plan.

Many resources on protein intake will equate a certain amount of protein per pound of your current weight. One popular range of consumption is .5 gram to 1 gram of protein per pound of weight each day, pending the exercise level. When I started my current program, I came in at 166 pounds, so the range was 83 to 166 grams of protein daily.

While you are vetting your protein intake, consider the various sources of protein that are most common in the modern American diet. Most common will be meats, but there are also grains, dairy and green leafy vegetables that will provide protein content.

I think this will be an appropriate time to share some personal information. I have been a vegetarian for the past 13 years. I don't have a platform I'm promoting, or any religious or political statements to make. It fits for me but I am not suggesting it's necessarily for you.

I'd suggest you work from your current diet and modify pieces and parts, using a gradual transition and test results as you go. Remember, this is a fluid, moving experiment over the course of time. We aren't in a hurry; we're going to be deliberate and plan to be successful.

The only person you have to ask about change is you. You're becoming well-versed through reading and research, so why not rest secure in the fact that the best nutrition decisions are the ones you thoughtfully execute.

My program sources most of its protein through custom smoothies, in pre-packaged fitness bars, and through meatless products (DISCLAIMER: I am not a medical doctor. This is my personal opinion on protein intake. Please see your health care professional prior to making any personal diet changes or modifications).

I love smoothies, but they have to taste good. Take a few moments to check the various sources of powdered protein. You'll identify dairy sources such as whey (from the cheese making process) and casein (from milk). Some sources are fast-burn, others digest more slowly. You'll also note plant based proteins from soybean and others from hemp, peas or brown rice.

Some brands of soy protein that mix well and have a great vanilla taste. Most provide 25 grams of protein per scoop; mix it with a cup of fruit, your favorite flavor of powdered drink mix mixed with water (I like cherry pomegranate) and blend. My smoothies are good enough that I can forego ice cream and frozen yogurt, rather waiting until I get home for one of these 180 calorie treats.

In the Mind over Diet tradition, keep reading and researching your protein plans. Several articles surfaced that estrogen-like compounds found in soy proteins can cause "man boobs" and other possible man-function issues. It may not be scientifically confirmed, but I transitioned my protein to a balance of soy on some days and plant-based protein on other days. There are some fine hemp, pea and chia seed blends that taste fabulous mixed with almond milk and frozen fruit.

In order to keep things convenient and fast, I buy big bags of frozen fruit for my smoothies; my favorites are mangos, tropical mix or mixed berries. Frozen fruit keeps the smoothies icy cold without having to add ice cubes and dilute the mix. With my high powered blender, I can mix my smoothies in a very thick consistency. Some of the body builder types call this "sludge" but I'd suggest Mind over Diet proponents can do better than that! Let's consider our thick smoothie mix a substitute for the ice cream. My thick drinks are so good that I'm able to forego ice cream or frozen yogurt and instead make my own dessert at home.

Here's some information to file in your schema. Do you frequent the new self-serve frozen yogurt stores? Are you opted for some of the add-on toppings? Not only are they expensive, but a large cup can rack up 500-600 calories. Weigh that against a whole blender of super smoothie mix with a whopping 50 grams of pure protein, at about 250 calories and no fat. Is that choice hard to make? When you understand and engage the content, you'll be moving towards a deeper understanding and take control of your own plan. In Mind over Diet, no one is telling you what to eat, or when to eat it. You're in charge, you've done the work, and you understand the foundation that is necessary to succeed.

Powdered protein has become a multi-million dollar industry, so be aware that marketers abound. There are many additives that are incorporated into protein, so you will be scrutinizing the pros and cons of brands, which include compounds, purity, taste and a consideration always important to me – cost.

Concocting great smoothies with appropriate protein content is an art. One new twist in the process are "super blenders" which are high watt and can turn most anything into liquid. I treated myself to a new model over the Christmas holiday and it's a game changer. Maybe it's a man and power tools thing, but when that monster roars it's exciting!

I have learned to enhance my traditional smoothie mix with whole carrots, red cabbage, celery and kale. Certain veggies can add an earthy taste to the mix, but I am improvising and gaining a new appreciation for what my blender can produce.

When you're traveling or don't have access to a blender or the goods to produce a full blown smoothie, you can resource and purchase pre-packaged protein drinks. These little containers can pack 30 grams of high-octane whey protein, have low sugar, and come in at around 160 calories. The taste isn't bad and you're getting the content needed to fuel both muscles and hunger.

During the day, I nibble through several high protein energy bars. Some deliver as much as 30 grams of protein, but beware that the "big" bars can also come in at over 400 calories. I consider these bars as meal replacement rather than snack. But, that's rather easy for me, as I don't often eat meals. Rather, it's grazing or sipping smoothies.

When I do opt for meals, I have become partial to meat substitute products. Some of these meatless wonders are so good I had to check the pack twice to make sure I wasn't eating meat! There are pseudo-sausage brands that deliver 26 grams of protein. I like to make a large tossed salad and set a grilled sausage on top for eating pleasure. Other meat-like products are soy based in burger form, while others use black beans as a foundation. We will discuss preparation in detail a bit later, but I like to cook my burgers to a sizzle hot state in a small electric grill that heats on both the top and bottom.

If you choose to consume meat, plan time to research where your meat originates. There is a cost-versus-value proposition in all products and meat is no exception. Do a bit of reading on growth hormones and antibiotics that are part of the beef and poultry process. It's an issue. A new alternative has emerged, through animals that are grass fed and free range, free of additives. However, you will pay a premium price for specialized meat. The origin of meat is a big debate in diet and fitness circles; Mind over Diet says you'll become informed and make your own decision.

You'll find some protein in grains and vegetables, but those sources may not provide enough grams per day to meet your total requirements. Your challenge is to project your daily protein needs then find optimum combination to meet those needs.

I like to discuss protein sourcing first, because my greatest success has originated in the process of sourcing ample protein into my daily diet, then following with limited carbs. If you're eating clean sources of protein and carbs, most all of the fat will be derived from preferable sources. Eat clean and ingest good fats; eat processed and fast foods and ingest fat that congeals in your veins and slides onto your love handles.

The procurement of carbs come next. Some carbs work better than others and the key indicator is how much sugar – natural or not – in laced into the food product.

**Research carb intake and determine the proper amount of carbohydrates per day, per pound of body weight.**

I love fruit, but fruit carries fructose and when I get too much, its affects my insulin. Mind over Diet isn't a science reporting effort so we won't go too deep here, but understand that when you ingest sugar you can produce insulin spikes. Fast burn/high glycemic carbs give a rush of energy, but then a crash. Ever have those days when you can't keep your head off the desk? I'd suggest that your food intake prior to the crash was high glycemic content. Understand the difference between fast burn and slow burn carbs. A good standardized measure is the glycemic index of foods. Eating low glycemic product is good on most occasions.

Knowing your protein and where you will source it lets you take command of your Mind over Diet program. Not only is protein a slow burn product in itself, it can also lessen the insulin spike you might get from fructose (sugar in fruit) or other higher glycemic carbs. Match your protein in combo with carbs and you'll lessen the sugar effect and also keep your engine burning clean.

Some examples of "good carbs" are the lower glycemic fruits such as apples, cherries or grapefruit. For vegetables consider asparagus, broccoli or celery. Another option is sweet potatoes as part of a nice mix with other veggies. Clean eating is related to clean cooking. It can remain rather simple, as I throw most everything in the steamer.

Information on high and low glycemic foods is readily available; there are small booklets to review, or numerous internet sources to investigate. Remember that in almost all cases, data is not hard to find. It's the individual who is engaged in Mind over Diet who searches out that data and utilizes it in daily planning.

There are some simple considerations that may help as you develop your Mind over Diet nutrition plan. Frozen vegetables are known to retain much of their nutrients. They are pre-packaged in single serving bags and are a great value. Frozen veggie stir fry mixes less than two dollars and mixed vegetables are even less. Much of my eating plan isn't fancy, but rather practical based on the food sources I know need to be in my body. Steam a bag of frozen vegetables, add a grilled black bean burger, add a dash of spice and you're putting your fork to a good balance of carbs and protein. That proves to be simple but effective.

Another big consideration is consumption of grains. This food source is evident in many items such as cereals, breads and pastas. Some common grain-based products are oatmeal, popcorn, rye bread, tortillas and brown or white rice.

Grain consumption has been controversial. You'll read more on that in just a moment. Many sources, including government health agencies, have long promoted portions of grain based food as a good and essential dimension of our diets. Other factions have now linked grains to carbs and eventually to fat conversion. Grains have also recently been linked to gluten and many individuals are identifying gluten as causing an allergic reaction.

Consider how you will approach the grain debate. I have cut back on most all breads and pastas, but still enjoy some grains in their essential forms. One of my favorite snacks is hot cereal. I enjoy rice, quinoa, 7-grain including flax seed, and of course old fashioned oatmeal. If you do the research and decide some amount of grains are good for you, brown rice isn't too expensive and makes a good base with veggies.

Here's another simple "cheater" treat I love, sometimes when I plan to stay in at night and want something to come close to dessert. I whip up a hot batch of waffles. I'm not eating bread, donuts or other dough-based foods, so my waffle jag is the closest I get to that category of goodies.

Let me put a new spin on your waffle intake. No syrup, no butter, nothing on top at all. They become hot, low calorie pastries, hot out of the waffle maker.

Here's how it's done: Buy a "complete" version of pancake and waffle mix...that means all you need to add is water. I like to mix my batter in a mixing cup. No precise measurements, just put about 1.5 cups of waffle mix in the cup, add water and mix until the consistency is slightly on the thin side. Then, stir in a few scoops of sweetener. I use an artificial sweetener and that too is controversial (more to come on that soon). I must admit I like sweet, so I had about three heaping tablespoons.

Heat your waffle maker to high; I like to grease mine with a spray of olive oil just before I pour in the batter. Let the mix hit the griddle and cook for about two minutes. You should extract a light, fluffy, hot treat. I eat mine like finger food, just pull a piece off and let it melt in your mouth!

My waffle recipe isn't a bad infraction on the calorie column, but it will rank high in the carb column. You can have two or three medium size waffles for about 320 calories. When you are planning to be a long term Mind over Diet devotee, it's important to innovate. Think outside the box and create treats that aren't too bad for the body and that satiate your desire for treats that aren't too detrimental.

I believe it's more valid to have gas in the tank that I enjoy over trying to achieve the "perfect" diet that will (attempt to) achieve improved performance and weight loss. Knowledge is power and improvising your Mind over Diet plan is a healthy process. Enjoy engaging the process. Part of schema shift is engaging an ongoing lifestyle process.

We aren't trying to be miserable until we reach some fabricated end result. Mind over Diet isn't hitting a specific weight goal and ending the process. Mind over Diet is reaching and aspiring to something new, better and more well developed that what we were attempting in the week or month prior.

Continue to grow and realize that you are capable of assimilating information and coming to your own conclusions. Media and marketing sources many times promote food products, recipes and supplements. Instead, think in terms of protein, carbs, and fats in your overall caloric intake. It's a Mind over Diet shift in schema, understanding the source of content and steering around what the food is "wrapped" in.

It is important to stay aware of what I call "trigger additives" in your food analysis. For me, that comes in the form of sugar (or sugar replicators), salt and bad oils in the form of preparation, such as deep fat frying. If I don't manage in these areas, these additives can trigger my inner addict. We can alter and shuffle the files in our schemas, but nonetheless some of the old files do remain. Return to the same bad behaviors and these negative and repetitive action files will resurface.

For example, I can go too deep into sucralose sweetener. I love it on oatmeal, in my waffles, in tea and on sweet potatoes. Although this product is zero calories, it promotes a craving for more, and "more" bring my calories count past optimal on that given day. Salted nuts are also a potential binge food. A lesser evil is French fries or other fried foods, but I still remain aware of the potential to overdo it. It's usually possible to note when these negative events are occurring, because your mind will start searching for the files that will support a rationalization for the ongoing ingestion of trigger additives.

While planning your eating plan, consider the density of the foods you will ingest. Good health, well-being and weight loss are all associated with a clean digestive tract. We want our bodies to digest the foods we eat, assimilate the valuable nutrients, and then purge the remainder as waste. What we don't want is a backup in the system.

Consider what can happen if you're eating predominantly dense foods. If you push a steady stream of meat, cheese and assorted fats into your stomach, the body takes from 24 to 72 hours to move those products completely through the digestive tract. If you pile in additional dense foods prior to the processing time, you may become backed up, with impacted feces in the colon.

I don't think there's any more need for more detail. But consider this: Why do you think there are so many cleanse diets popping up in your research? Obesity has a link to less than optimum processing systems. That's an image to hold onto when you are eating fruits and vegetables as dominant over meats and fats. As a Mind over Diet advocate, I'm not about to set your standards for you, but will certainly encourage you to think about how much water, and fiber, your chosen foods contain.

The intended result is a system that purges clean and fast. When you identify different sources of protein, carbs and fats, you'll be able to also analyze density and make your own decision on popular diets that are in the ads and on the news.

Based on your personal research, you'll start seeing food in a different perspective. For example, I love eating huevos rancheros at my favorite Mexican restaurant. But when I look at the added chips, flour tortillas, cheese and all the add-ons, it's almost a day's worth of calories and an out-of-proportion fat intake. Please know I still enjoy that meal, but I understand the content and what I am ingesting.

Sourcing fresh food products is a special consideration. Some adhere to a "grow local, buy local" approach to foodstuffs. Other may be price conscious and do their produce shopping at a large chain grocer. There is also growth in area farmer's markets and what has become in some areas a trendy, yuppie, social event. Others are attempting to keep prices down so the lower and middle-classes can afford produce. You may be an environmentally aware citizen who is engaged with the local economy and holds a preference over food sourcing.

I realize this is the start of something good, but we have to find a way to get into our revised eating plans without emptying our wallets. We all have to adapt as it's comfortable. So I'm suggesting you can have your cake (kale?) and eat it too, if you shop and buy wisely.

The Mind over Diet plan will require plenty of fresh, clean food, so these are personal considerations you will need to address. I'm a mix and match food-source individual. Sometimes I buy from the big chain grocers, at other times from our local health food chain, and yet on other occasions from the local farm market or local produce vendor. We can all make choices on when and how we shop and I plan to stay aware of cost vs. value vs. economic impact to my community.

Now that you have worked to identify and source different foods that work in your Mind over Diet plan, there are interesting considerations regarding the combinations and suggested volumes of food groups. I wanted you to explore and consider your own proportional intake before we moved to the next step, which is taking on the thousands of diet plans being promoted in today's marketplace.

**Use your search engine to explore "fitness diets" or "weight loss diets."**

Be prepared to engage thousands of sources regarding what foods are optimal for weight loss, muscle growth and fat loss. You'll find many passionate approaches to the best foods and the best combinations of food groups. There are advocates for the all fruit diet, the all meat-and-cheese diet, juicing diets, and a proportional mix of predominant protein to lesser but equal proportions of carbs and fats. You'll see dozens of sources purporting that they have definitive answers to health, nutrition, and weight loss. What's a consumer to do?

A great saying is, "you can't know where you're going, if you don't know where you've been." That surely applies to what has been construed and promoted as good dieting in years past. Most all of us have been exposed to the original "food pyramid" that indicates our daily intake should be 6-11 servings of cereal, rice and pasta; 3-5 servings of vegetables; 2-3 servings of dairy products; 2-3 servings of meat; and a limited amount of fats, oil and sweets.

On the athletic front, I can remember years of recommendations to "carb up." Anyone what connected with the running community can remember the huge spaghetti dinners that were presented as precursors to major city marathons. The memory sticks in my mind, thousands upon thousands of runners, all gorging on plate after plate of pasta on the eve of the event. At that point we believe it was a necessity, that without the carbs for fuel model, we'd never make it to the finish line!

You'll also note diets that advocate for foods prepped vs. non-prepped. The raw food diet has its followers, those who belief the energy and power of food comes through its natural state. I recall one diet book for weight loss that was 90% or more raw vegetables on salads. I have gone down that path and over time, raw became not palatable for me. Maybe I was just over crunching, but a nice mix of veggies lightly steamed with some seasoning goes across the tongue and down to the belly in a more friendly fashion.

If you're similar to me, it's nice to start an analysis with a visual overview. For an interesting Mind over Diet exercise, run an Internet search for "food pyramid" and then hit the images tab. It's actually difficult to find the traditional food model because a multitude of new variations are available. Consider the nutrient dense pyramid, the raw food pyramid, the "real food" pyramid, or the new MyPlate.gov pyramid, which proposes fairly equal portions of fruits, grains, and protein, with a slight emphasis on vegetables and dairy as a satellite and less consumed food group.

As you peruse your Internet content, you're sure to come upon a diet and exercise package that has emerged into a culture, predominantly driven by modern high intensity workout routines. A major "brand" in this movement is the Paleo diet. This plan is based on our Paleolithic ancestors who lived in the hunter-gatherer mode. Paleo advocates adhere to the finest non-modified sources for meat, low glycemic vegetables, low consumption of fruit, no grains, and good fats. One example of a Paleo concoction is a big chunk of butter stirred into "bullet proof" coffee.

The Paleo diet crowd many times suggests fasting for short periods. It is believed this is advantageous, for that is how our ancestors survived. No hunting success on a given day – no eating that night. Paleo dieters see grains as something that was manufactured by humans and that grains do not have origins in a natural state. There's an addendum to this discussion, in that much of wheat, soy and corn products grown today and produced in a genetically modified state.

Paleo advocates sometimes state that it's not about calorie counting, but rather the meat/good carb/good fat content. This is where the Mind over Diet plan suggests vetting these theories, considering for yourself what is necessary and how you will negotiate your personal eating plan.

I personally came upon some cognitive dissonance over the Paleo diet. Since I am a vegetarian, I searched for options within food parameters that might suit my own convictions. Bottom line, I fell off into a cheddar cheese cube and almond diet and gained about 12 pounds. That's wasn't my intended outcome, but it is a result of the "calories don't count" mentality I tried to embrace.

However, one big schema shift I encountered by studying Paleo wasn't in the diet, it was in the relationship between the diet and related exercise. Paleo fans many times state their exercise base in minimal, that the ripped tone of their bodies is due to the proper intake of protein and fat over bad carbs.

I've been formulating thoughts the past several days, wrapping my brain around health, wellness, fitness, exercise, objectives and outcomes. It's almost too much to explicate over a 10-mile run, but I'll do my best to bring you some fresh observations.

What set me off was the nutrition world's heightened awareness of all things Paleo. If you haven't yet jumped on the Paleo bandwagon, it's about eating like a cave man, from an era when hunting and foraging was predominant over farming. Bottom line, it's focused on lean meats, vegetables leaning towards the green variety, with minimal fruits, nuts and oils. Grains were thrown under the bus, along with most all dairy derivatives.

My schema took me in a different direction. It was the "eat now, burn it off later" mentality. I was into big miles on the bike and running and in my schema exercise was the focus, more than the quality of the fuel I was eating. Have you ever seen a runner polish off a pizza and several beers, then state "don't worry, I'll run it off later."

Here's a secret. Over the Christmas holiday, I was running 10 miles a day, every day, and was gaining weight. I fell off the bandwagon and my holiday eating was getting the best of me. Poor food choices can quickly win the race over amount of exercise. We'll speak more about this in the fitness section of this book.

I may have spun out on cheese and almonds, but my learning outcome was quite profound. Set your personal standards, eat well, and your exercise can become realistic and enjoyable. Food choices are a priority and your journey into dozens of diets will help you form your own master plan. Your takeaways may be different from mine, but they are nonetheless just as valid. Processing the alternative points of view allow you to become informed and intelligently engage the debate.

Your research may lead to those who adhere to a complete vegetarian diet. The strictest adherence to vegetarianism is defined by the vegan diet.

Veganism is the purest form of vegetarian eating; it's free of all dairy sources and for most, it's sourced from organic fruits and vegetables. Being a vegan is quite difficult, as foods that are not self-prepared must come under scrutiny. Consider eating at a restaurant: Were the veggies cooked in animal fat derived oil? Was my serving "contaminated" by touching a spoon that came in contact with meat?

Vegan dieters are proponents of the wide ranging benefits that are manifested in this pure form of eating. There are theories that veganism assists in healing, offers a performance boost for athletics, and can regenerate the mind. Some approach a vegan lifestyle as a form of religion, connecting food to the optimum body and mind experience.

If you become enthralled with going fruit and veggie all the way, other realities can hit home. There may be cost and affordability issues. All one has to do is source some of the recommended products at your local health food store and it's clear you might need a second job to afford this style of eating; have you priced Chia seeds lately?

You may run into diets that don't tell you what to eat, but rather what not to eat. One popular variation is the "no sugar" diet; just get rid of the sweets and all will be exceptional in your life. When considering this, please recall that fructose in a form of sugar in fruit. Start cutting sugar, start cutting fruit and you may find your food plan is no longer satisfying.

Some diets will try to transition its adherents from low carb to no carb. I know a successful fitness trainer and body builder who has won regional competitions by reducing all carbs out of her diet. She was "cut" to the maximum but in the end it wasn't sustainable. In my last conversation with this motivated individual, she (and her dog) had transitioned to a vegan diet.

Her comment of "I did it before, I know how to do it again" is predictive of what many diets that produce the images we see in magazines and on the web. Unless it's a full time occupation and part of your job, sustaining the body fat/muscle ratio necessary to be "shredded" is not for the rank and file consumer. You may have best intentions, but sometimes life and related choices may get in the way. That's why preparation and planning on your own terms will be viable, over mandates to "eat this" or "don't eat that."

What's interesting about the no carb diet is that it is an end to a goal, but one that does not seem sustainable. If you're one who can live on chicken breasts and cottage cheese, you may be in for the long haul. But as a Mind over Diet master planner, you may want to develop an outline for eating that is sustainable and attractive as part of your lifestyle.

When designing your Mind over Diet eating routine and exploring the marketing at hand, make sure to study condiments, dressings and other flavor enhancers. A few tablespoons of condiments can add hundreds of calories to what was a nutritious plate of food. Some experts will promote olive oil as a wonderful additive to your foods and diet. I'm an olive oil fan, but under the pretense that there's

119 calories in one tablespoon. If you liberally pour olive oil over your salad you may add 1000 calories!

Try seasonings and spices, but don't overdo the sodium. My favorite spices bring a zing to most anything I'm eating. I keep several flavors in the cabinet so that, in rotation, there's a variation in the taste of my foods.

More greens always seem to be a good addition to any diet. You might find some sources who propose an all salad diet (I've actually seen books written on it) but that can be hard to sustain. You may have charged into salad eating in the past, only to hit salad burnout. This is a personal Mind over Diet decision. If you can keep a big salad on the table and eat it each day, I'd forge ahead.

If salads aren't your thing, consider my prior comments on how to liquefy greens in a smoothie. I have almost tripled my greens intake since moving to a high power blender. I hope the results show from that shift in overall lifestyle. Kale is getting high ratings and some suggest throwing a few leaves into the blender with a smoothie. Other vegetables that can be readily assimilated into your blender mix include raw cabbage, spinach, green apples (contributes tartness and sweetness) or green, red and yellow peppers.

As you expand your knowledge base, you'll be making daily choices on both food types and also food preparation. There are some go-to options I'd like you to consider. Several manufacturers produce 100 calorie bags of microwave popcorn. There are butter, kettle corn, and other variations that you will find appealing. It's a nice amount of fluffy food and you're locked at just 100 calories. Not many snacks come in that low. For example, I grabbed a bag of trail mix the other day and cleaned it off, then looked later and noted I had ingested almost 1200 calories!

It's no secret fruit is a popular option. I realize that too much fructose (fruit sugar) isn't a good thing, but fruit in moderation is part of every day of my life. When you clean up your diet, you'll learn to appreciate the natural sweet taste of oranges, apples, bananas, grapes, etc. It's good nutrition going into your body with a low calorie outcome.

A quick and complete meal can be found in steamed brown rice and vegetables. I have a two-stage steamer and place brown rice on the lower level with a load of vegetables on top. Most of the time 50 minutes is appropriate and you're ready for a steaming plate of non-processed food. The calorie count is low and fiber content (in brown rice) is beneficial.

There are also many great hot cereal options. The gold standard is old fashioned oatmeal, but there are also multigrain cereals, brown rice cereals, wheat variations and also hot quinoa cereals. I like to add a bit of salt, microwave in a bowl in about 3 minutes, add a bit of sweetener and stir. You will enjoy a nice bowl and feel full for approximately 150 calories. On some days, I'll turn a bowl of hot cereal into a meal by adding some raisins or a banana.

We discussed smoothies, but think for a moment how smoothies can serve as a dessert, meal replacement of mid-day snack. If you're careful you can mix a low calorie combo with ingredients such as frozen fruit, zero calories powdered drink mix and protein. What's amazing is that you can produce a blender full – about three standard glasses – for less than 300 calories. It's rocket fuel after my workout each morning and serves as breakfast.

There are more foodstuffs you can integrate into your diet, but the ones above have really set the foundation for me. Add a few energy bars each day and you're on the way to being ripped and ready for your upcoming endurance sport season.

As you develop your refreshed schema, be sure to stay alert and keep aware of the food types and related calorie values that will cross your path. I remember a time when I was taking my elderly father (now deceased) out for a few errands. On the way home, I had promised him a treat. He's been a chocolate malt lover for many years, so we stopped on the way back to his apartment. I grabbed a small chocolate for him, but also succumbed to point-of-sale advertising and ordered a large flavored shake for myself.

I enjoyed every sip of that delectable concoction, until it was time to enter it into my calorie counter system. It shocked me with a whopping 770 calories! It was good, but never good enough to warrant one third of what should have been my daily caloric intake. Remember that when bad food choices like large shakes enter into the equation, there are no magic potions or 10-minute-a-day workouts that will negate those food decisions.

It's possible to isolate your food management, planning and decision-making. Here are a few points that can assist in putting healthy products in the engine and fight the battle of the bulge.

Get some distance from food. Step way back and examine it from afar. It's not your friend and in most cases it can prove to be the enemy. Food is not entertainment, but food can be incorporated into the social experiences you will encounter. It's important to make that psychological paradigm shift, in that food is peripheral to, but not the object of, your fun and satisfaction. You can't base friends and fun around a meal. Go out to eat and maintain a heightened awareness that there's a much greater probability you'll make the wrong choices. Many options in a restaurant are way off your eating goal, so be aware of that.

Food is not a drug that is used to satiate the senses and dull our emotions. Eating as a hobby is out. This is huge challenge in my personal journey. I love to graze and hit the cupboards every ten minutes in the evenings. This is where mindful eating comes in. Face the truth; 90% of the time when you want to eat, you aren't hungry. Matter of fact, start to note when you are actually hungry. My experience indicated that I was ingesting food to offset boredom or to satiate my taste buds, or to get a sugar rush. However, eating to curb hunger was a rare occurrence.

See all foods as calories. A long, consistent use of your exercise and food app will get you to the place where you know the cost of calories vs. a food choice. Snacking on a 100 calorie bag of popcorn may make sense, but that big dish of ice cream at 9 pm may dump 500+ calories into your gut. It comes down to simple math, calories in (food) and calories out (exercise and activity).

Please read and digest these recommendations and put a positive spin in the revelations. I realize that this may paint a bleak picture, but it's not meant to. It's about delayed gratification; you can get the immediate rush of a food binge or you can wait over time to see that ripped physique in the mirror. The price to pay can be substantial (over your former life habits) but the outcome associated with your Mind over Diet plan will offer great rewards. With Mind over Diet, you can get in the game or stay on the sidelines; it's your choice and mine.

There's one additional dimension I'd like you to address. It's bound to come into play as you work through your Mind over Diet transformation. It surely has jolted me as I go through the process of carving off those last few pesky pounds. It has happened to me during several weight loss periods – the set point barrier.

In the set point model, our bodies have a control system that dictates how much fat each of our human shells should carry. This theory (and I'll call it that, because it's up to you to consider its merit) contends we are born with either a high or low fat setting - it wasn't up to you. No one knows how to change that inherent setting and no matter what we attempt, we will revert to that prior constant weight the set point keeps your weight fairly constant.

Weight loss efforts many times deliver a quick initial loss of poundage, but then the effort plateaus, despite ongoing exercise and diet efforts. The theory states that your body knows its optimum weight and fat set point. Some also argue that if you move too far below your set point, you may find a decrease in a stable, optimistic mood. Push the set point down and depression and lethargy can follow.

So where do we go from here? The set point advocates state that as we drop pounds our set point bodies push the metabolic rate even lower. Dieting becomes less effective and further weight loss is almost impossible. I might consider some of the points made regarding set point, but I'd also interject several variables that may demonstrate how you can break a set point and move to a different plateau.

Let your strong mind control the body. We are given great brains and they have power to establish constraints. Feed your engine with positive weight loss messaging. Meditate on your new set point and why it will be beneficial to arrive there.

It's also possible to shock the system. For me, that was breaking out of the 90-minute run routine and turning it into a 10+ mile routine. Now mileage is not dependent on time, instead time is dependent on mileage. If you're stuck in the lack of progress mode, try some changes to your Mind over Diet plan.

Calories do count. Some modern programs discount this, but I'll strongly suggest that if you have a 4000 calorie workout day, then eat 2000 calories on that day, some body composition changes will be in store (if you replicate this sort of day on regular occasion).

When your body goes through a transition and you are feeding it with clean, non-processed food, you'll earn a change up in composition – less fat pounds, more muscle pounds. That's why I like to track body fat on my home scale. It helps me measure my weight change in relation to the positive or negative trending in body fat. When your body is building muscle, it burns clean food more efficiently and you can use the change in body composition to fight past a set point.

Stay conscious of your journey and lean into the head knowledge you've created. Your new, revised schema is a powerful tool and you need to use it to rationalize and adapt to each phase of your Mind over Diet program. I face the fact I'm in some instances, I'm in a challenging place with weight loss and fitness. If I'm stuck on a set point, I get scientific. I weigh each morning after my workout and log the stats. I take my blood pressure each morning and evening. I look at my running output, with downloads into my computer from my GPS watch. Some of my favorite metrics are average pace per mile and average heart rate for each session. When I stay highly connected to the stats, I can make decisions on what to change and how to make those changes.

As part of breaking the set point, I'll sometimes shake up the food intake. Set a base calorie limit for the day, then experiment. I work with 2000 and try shifting my proteins, types of energy bars, when I eat fruit, late night snack content, etc. Whatever your norm is, break loose and tell your body changes are underway and there's nothing it can do to stop the revolution.

This is not an easy journey. But if you commit, it's possible to experience change. When I started this crazy path in life in 1983, I was a long-time 213 pounds. I broke it down and reduced to 165. Now, over 30 years later, I weigh 165. I have stripped myself down to 153 on two occasions, but have not been able to hold that minimalist physique. Food binges, holidays and other difficult periods in life can shift the poundage up and then it's time to start clearing the mind for another recalibrating and recharge.

I'd like to encourage you in how the Mind over Diet effort can change your set point and bring you to a new place in life. My body is becoming light and crisp and in opposition to the theory, my mind is expanding and confident. There is a serene disposition that envelops me and I rest in the knowledge that I am fueling my body with clean, healthy food. If you're hanging a bit on the thick side, consider challenging your own set point. There's an amazing world on the other side.

Before we conclude this chapter, there's a multi-billion dollar industry we have yet to address, that of dietary supplements. It's based on what additions are needed to what we eat, what our food plan includes and if there are gaps we need to fill. Since many supplements are herbal in nature, they are not controlled by government agencies and many times purport to deliver amazing short cuts and accelerated results.

**Conduct an Internet search on "dietary supplements" and consider what a Mind over Diet researcher might add to a high performance meal plan.**

As with every other category, there are tons of options to consider. Do your joints hurt, or should you be preserving your joints? Take Glucosamine and/or Chondroitin. Are you deficient in vitamin A, or vitamin D?

Supplement immediately. How about making sure you're getting the proper levels of fatty acids? Maybe omega 3 fish oil is for you, or maybe omega 3-6-9, which is a combination of fish, borage and flax seed oils?

And if your sexual performance isn't at high wire status and you're a victim of erectile dysfunction, you can fix it with numerous "sexual nutrients" that are sure to please your significant other and demonstrate your prowess on any occasion.

The study and considerations for ingesting multivitamins are varied. This $28 billion industry provides special versions for all forms of consumers, for endurance sport athletes, body builders, yoga practitioners, and those products that differentiate female and male athletes. There are vitamins for the over 50 crowd, vitamins sorted into daily packs, vitamins that state they will help you memory, or vitamins that proclaim they will correct your vision.

Vitamin makers claim to increase your strength or aid in workout recovery. There are liquid vitamins, capsule vitamins, and powdered vitamins. Vitamins claim they will make you attack, or perform, or endure, or smile because you're happier after taking them.

The advantage to one (or now, in some cases, many) pills as a nutrient advantage is debatable. Take a vitamin pill on an empty stomach and much of its value will pass through your system and exit in the urine.

Recent studies by prominent media experts have reinforced the opinion that multivitamins deliver little, if any, value. These reports state that vitamins have no proven benefits and if taken if high dosages, may actually be harmful.

However, other experts within the vitamin manufacturing industry repute most of the claims, state that vitamins are safe. Some studies indicate health and performance gains.

It's an ongoing process to read and discover what makes sense for you. I have come to a less is better approach, but that's after years of taking a multivitamin, vitamin E, glucosamine and chondroitin, and at times some form of herbal fat burner mix. Reading leads to learning leads to a shift in our paradigms and a rebooted schema. I later learned I may need omega 3, but may be overdosed on omega 6 and omega 9. The buzz might be 3-6-9, but for me it's -6 and -9, just leave the 3!

What I find interesting about the supplement industry is that if you stay aware over time, it's a moving target. Ever hear of L-carnitine? Check it out. We called that substance the portal to getting "shrink wrapped" in the 1980's. Just recently I have been reading about Garcinia Cambogia Extract. That's another of the burn it off quicker additives. Want a better mood? You have to bump up your 5-HTP, ASAP!

There's surely some humor in this process, but my point is that each level of research will take you to another recommendation regarding yet another supplement. Be aware that for some, such as those in the body-builder population, supplements are a major consideration and can cost hundreds of dollars a month. I listen to one top endurance sport podcast where supplements are discussed on a regular basis. I'm in no way against the use of supplements and it's clearly a personal decision. But for me, cost and safety are paramount. In additional to racking up a big monthly expense, some supplements can be dangerous.

For example, ephedra was a popular additive to diet supplements several years ago, but it was found to have adverse effects and was banned in 2004. Geranium extract was also recently under scrutiny. It may have been called a "natural" stimulant, but cases of elevated blood pressure, shortness of breath and heart maladies were reportedly tied to the supplement.

Your heightened awareness will serve you well. Here's a tip: If you are attracted to slick advertising for a weight loss or fitness supplement, search for the ingredients and learn more about the active agents being marketed. Many times it's the package or the wrapper that draw the most attention. What's inside the bottle may be a common herbal mix, or in worse scenarios, a dangerous concoction you need to stay away from.

The more you engage the content of what goes into your body, the greater shift you'll earn in your schema. Also, your social identity will become more associated with the knowledge of nutrition, which will make you an advocate who can comment and suggest diet and training diet techniques for others.

However, beyond the content of supplements and their inherent value, consider the psychology inherent to the process of vetting these products. There's a heightened engagement that accompanies the exploration and discovery of the latest brands to hit the market. I buy much of my nutrition supplementation via the Internet, as I reside in a small community that many times does not offer my specific needs through local retailers. When one of my online providers launches a new line of fitness or weight loss items, I find motivation in reading and understanding the rationale behind the product and the active ingredients in the product.

The advantage may come from shuffling your supplement mix and bringing in a new product. That's where Mind over Diet works, in the sense you are adjusting your schema and achieving inspiration and a new step forward through awareness and change.

When you truly understand and control the content of food, you'll move off the set point (or stuck place) in body composition and step to the next level. At first, it seems like a strange place, as you won't be pseudo-fit, but rather lean and muscular. When you're eating clean, it's easier to hear your body ask for what it needs. That may be a protein rich plate of eggs with olive oil, or possibly a steaming bowl of old-fashioned oatmeal with honey. After running a hard 10 mile loop, I can sense my body yearning for the protein smoothie it will quickly digest and assimilate.

We all carry a history. It's possible to look in the rear view mirror and see the seasons of destruction, then the periods of care and rebuilding. If you're reading Mind over Diet, you're in a good place right now and are working to complement your lifestyle.

| | |
|---|---|
| Track all food ingested for one week; what is my average daily caloric intake? | _____ calories per day |
| Research recommended caloric intake per day for sedentary activity. Set your new calorie goals. | _____ calories per day |
| Research protein intake. How much, and what type of, protein should I ingest per pound of body weight each day? | _____ grams of protein |
| Research carbohydrate intake. How much, and what type of, carbs should I ingest per pound of body weight each day? | _____ grams of carbs |
| Research fats that are associated with your diet. What are "good" fats? How much fat will you consume each day? | _____ grams of fat |
| Based on target protein, carbs and total calories each day, define the types and amount of foods you will eat. | Devise food content list |
| What are your "trigger" additives? Where do they occur in your diet? | List "triggers" |
| How will your food allocation be distributed? What are your eating "touch points" throughout the day? | Schedule for consumption |

Developing a personal diet isn't perfect science. But this time around, I am confident your Mind over Diet plan will bring about the positive change needed for sustained performance and health.

*Chapter summary*

- Research and determine how many grams of protein (per pound of body weight) you'll target in your daily diet.

- Research and determine how many grams of carbohydrates (per pound of body weight) you'll target in your daily diet.

- Research the various sources of "clean" proteins and carbs and create a list of food products you will introduce into your diet.

- Beware of "trigger additives" and their potential to shift your schema to recurring negative eating habits.

- Research fitness diets. Determine what proportion of protein/carbs/fats you will target for your daily diet.

- Research dietary supplements promoted as part of your daily intake. Choose the essential mix of supplements that will complement your Mind over Diet nutrition blueprint.

# CHAPTER 6
## Fitness

My window of opportunity to finish a 100-mile ultrarun is closing quickly. I'm losing jogging speed and the will to suffer over a 28-hour span is not what is used to be. If I design a plan for making what might be my final attempt, the steps to get there will have to be something different.

A yoga instructor stated my "practice" is coming along well; when I complete one hour of forced stretching I feel invigorated. Swimming also unloads the legs and gives me a fresh, relaxed feeling. Being rested, pliable and non-injured has taken precedent over pounding out 70-mile weeks. There is a deep tiredness that comes into my body when I run too far, too fast, on too many days.

What are my recommendation for a training plan that can take a 50+ year old runner to a 100-mile ultradistance finish? I'd suggest it starts with:

- Focused diet, sub 2000 calories a day with all the right nutrients
- Easy-stroke one hour freestyle swim workout x 3/week

- Stretching one hour yoga sessions x 4/week

- Weight training/strength sessions x 3/week
- Mountain and road cycling sessions x 5/week
- Running at relaxed pace (10/min miles) x 3/week
- Commuter walking daily

Now that I have devised the plan with the highest potential, will it happen? It's not likely. This may be a viable route to success, but let's be real. There aren't many specimens out there who are 50+ and can traverse the 100-mile distance (within a mandatory 30 hour cutoff). For the select few masters' ultrarunners who remain, I'd suggest save the legs, eat fresh, get wet in the pool, and let your sensei be your guide.

I'm not suggesting that you're sharing my vision of a 100-mile run, but I wanted to kick off this chapter with an introduction on how the Mind over Diet process created a new outlook for my fitness planning.

For years I adhered to the "more is better" training technique. Of course that led to other complications, such as "blown legs" syndrome. That's an ultrarunner's malady that sets in when you have way too many miles on one's legs, miles that came with any reprieve for healing or recovery. That can cause chronic tiredness. Try lifting yourself off the couch, or climbing a flight of stairs. With a set of blown legs it's a challenge on each step of every day.

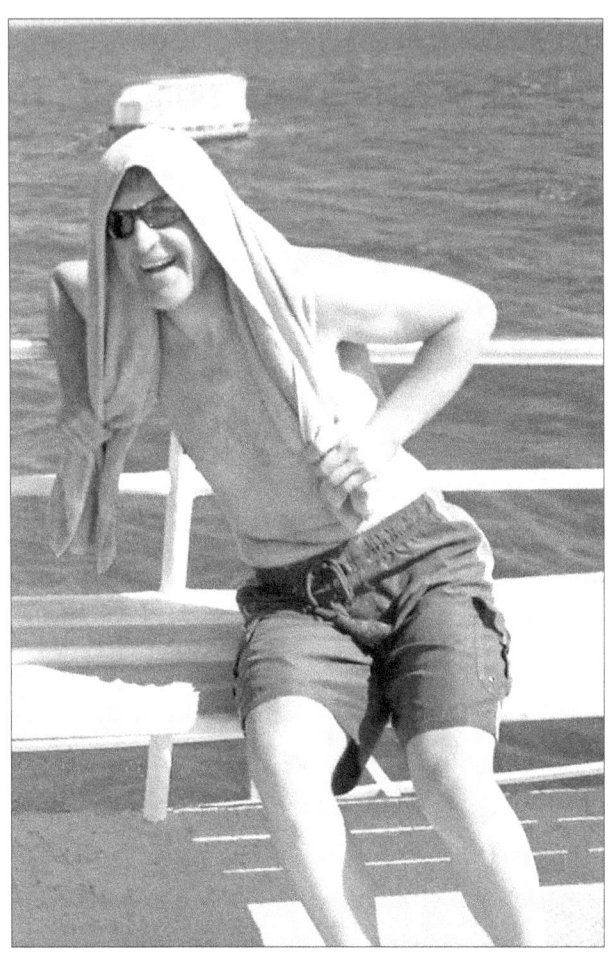

*My Mind over Diet journey has not been a perfect path. Here's an image from a prior summer vacation. My schema shifted and my predominant social identity was tied to overeating and food!*

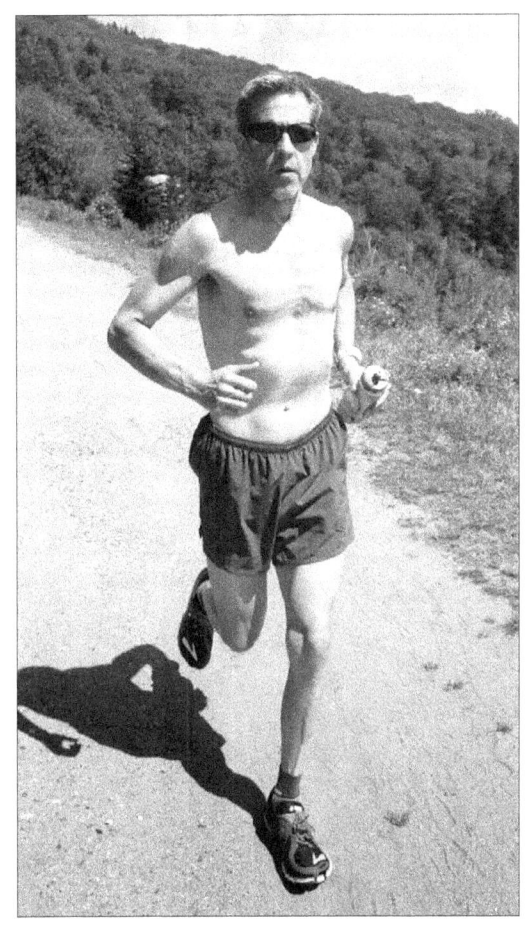

*My program took off after I reset my schema, refreshed my mind with the latest nutrition info, and reclaimed my social identity as an ultrarunner. This is 10 weeks after the previous picture.*

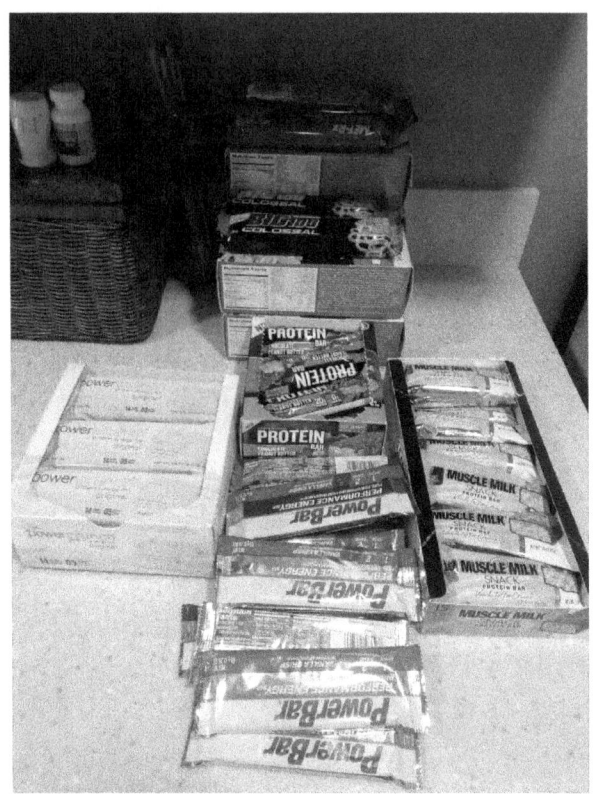

*There are several good options to ingest proteins and "good" carbs. I am a big adherent of energy bars. They are convenient and it's easy to know the exact proportion of nutrients.*

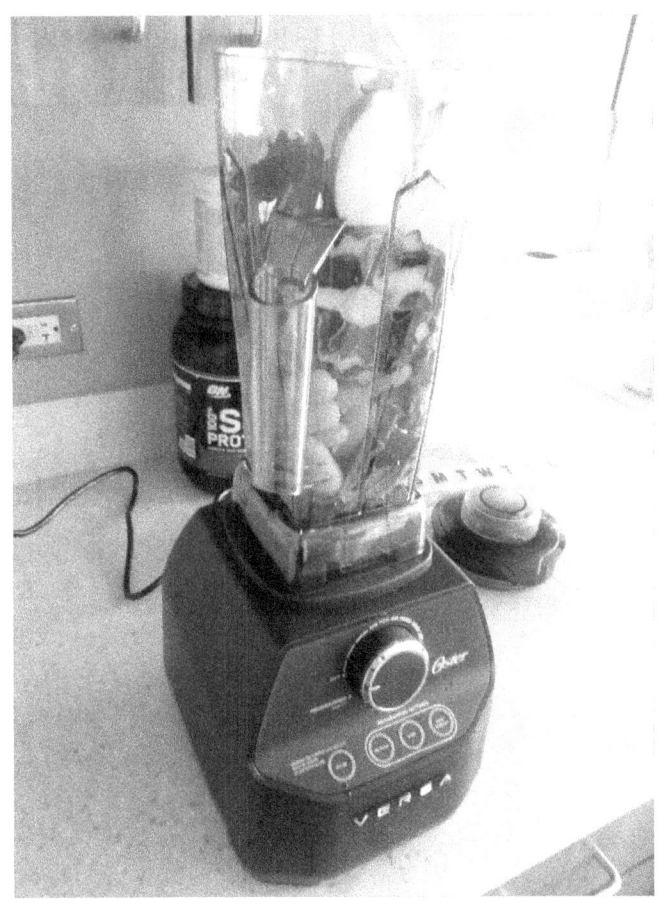

*If you want to push maximum rocket fuel into your system, try a high speed blender. Here's my kale, carrot, celery, red cabbage and green apple smoothie...with a few scoops of whey or soy protein.*

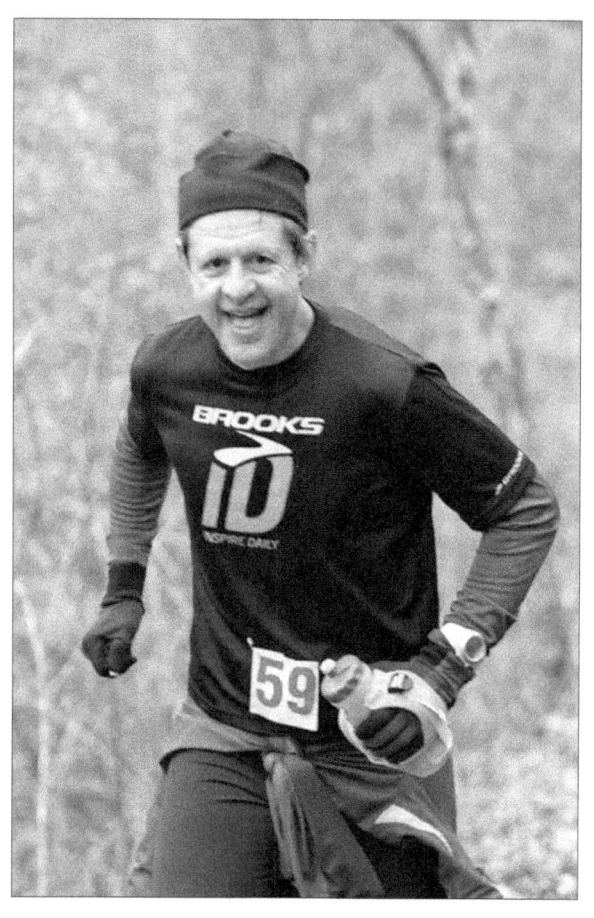

*It's the ultrarunner life. I have been running marathons, then ultradistance races, for over 30 years. Mind over Diet allows for the constant provisioning of attitude so that nutrition and fitness stay fresh and enticing.*

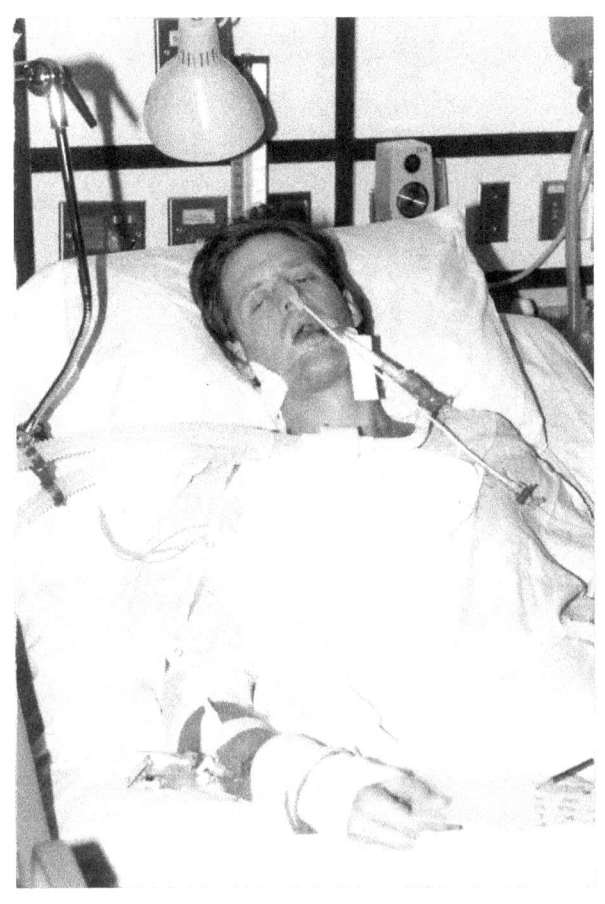

*Mind over Diet was partially created through my 1993 experience with Guillain-Barre Syndrome. Paralysis and the consequent rehabilitation taught me that psychological aspects are paramount to success.*

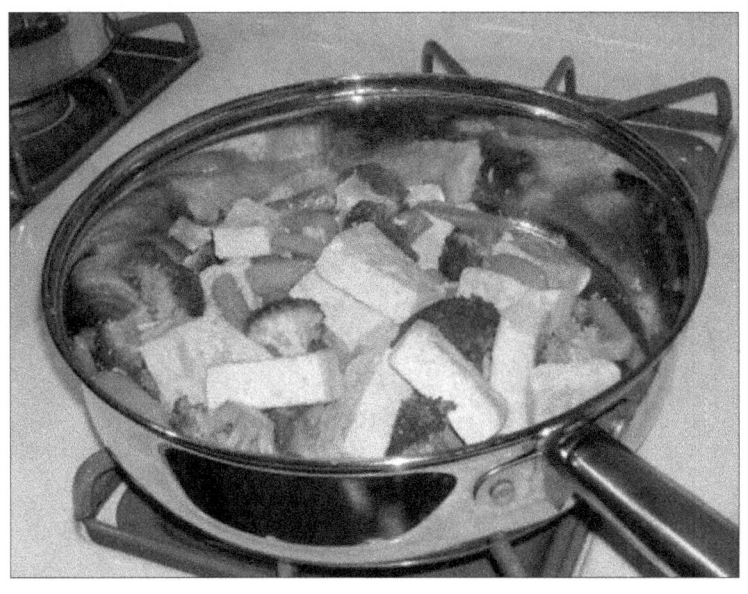

*Mind over Diet embeds your brain with the essentials in good nutrition, then helps you build your own plan. Here's a fresh veggie and tofu stir fry (grill tofu in olive oil, then add veggies, finally Szechuan sauce). This is my good protein/good carb favorite dinner.*

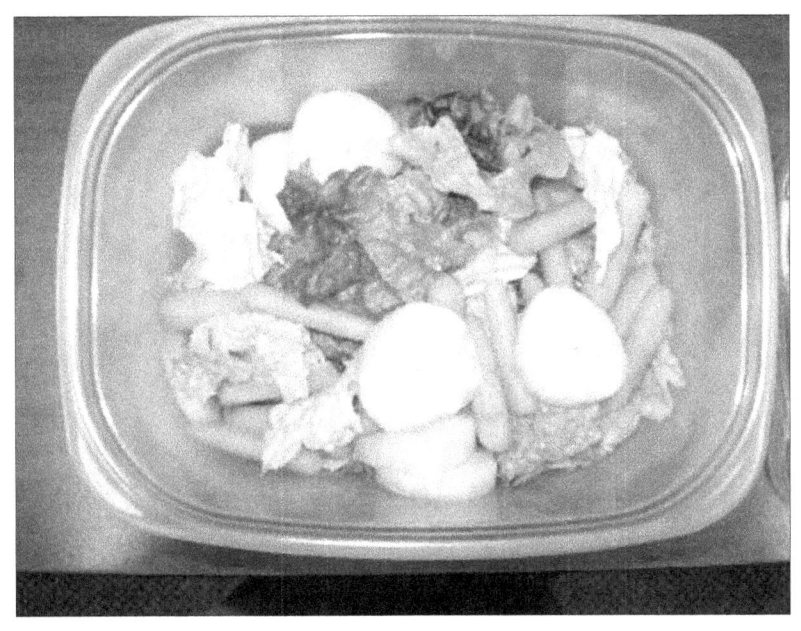

Does this seem boring? Maybe so but it's high fiber, low carb fuel that carries well and serves as a mid-day meal. I keep olive oil and seasoning and my office so I can prep the salad just prior to eating; that keeps it fresh and crunchy.

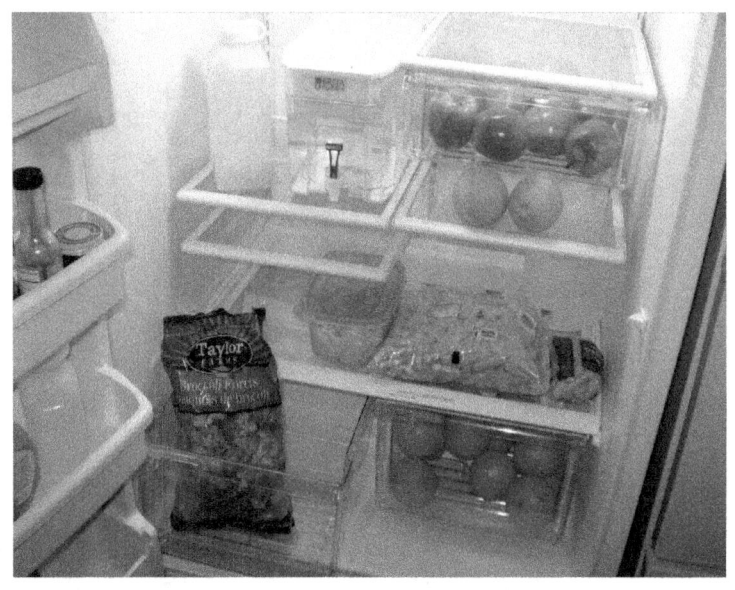

Here' an image of my fridge when things were prepped for optimum performance. It took several months of setting a new psychological perspective to reach this modified plateau. Clean eating also shifts one's social identity to an association with nutrition.

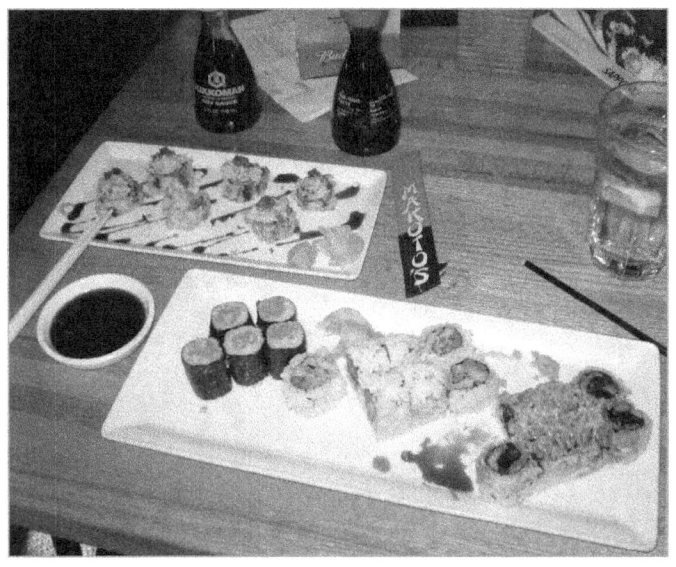

Is sushi on your menu? I like to eat a variety of rolls. If you're not into eating raw seafood, get rolls that are all veggie, or with cooked forms of fish. Sushi makes for a nutritious, non-processed meal.

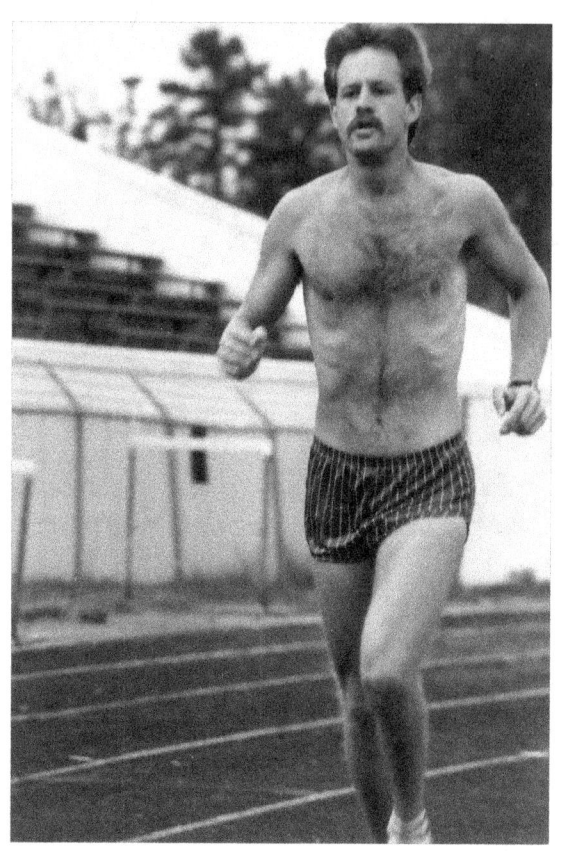

*Here's a shot of me circa 1986, running two six-minute miles as part of a Greensboro (NC) run club event. Mind over Diet is about longevity in planning, motivation and satisfaction in nutrition and fitness.*

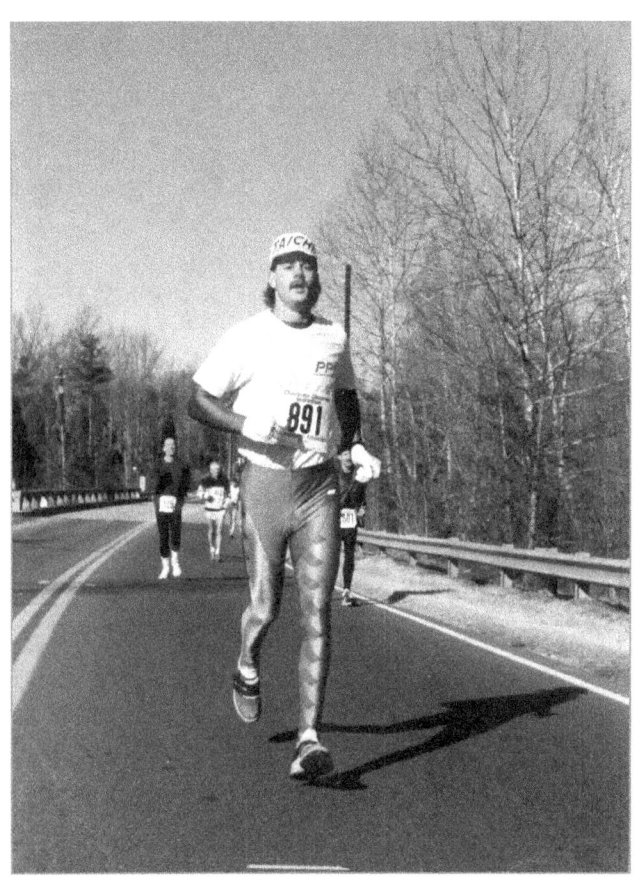

*I made great apparel choices in my first marathon, Charlotte in 1987. My social identity started as a triathlete, then marathon runner, then ultradistance finisher. Now, the Mind over Diet analysis has taken me into cycling, strength training and yoga.*

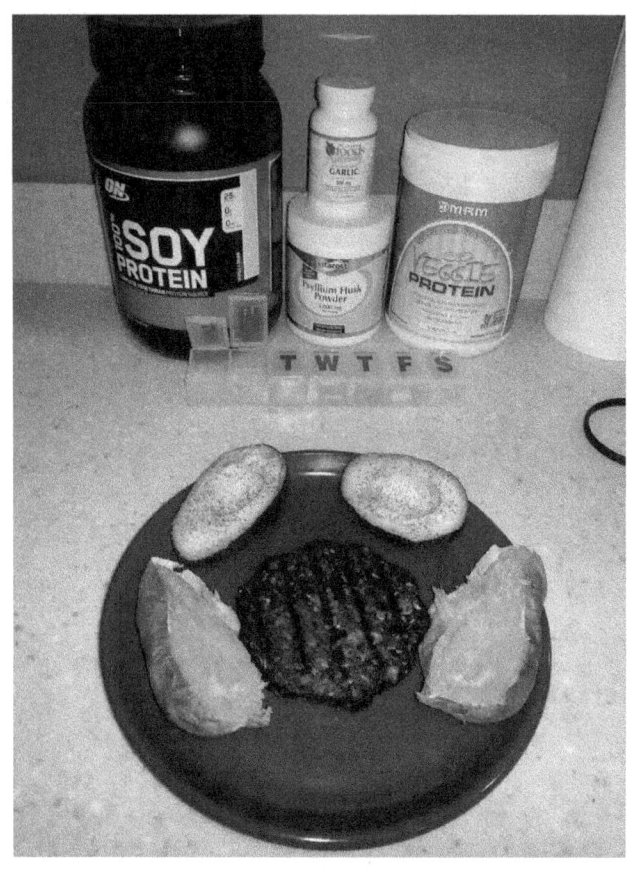

*Simple but effective: Here's a combo that serves as a low carb, slow burn nutrition meal. Consider avocado with spicy seasoning, grilled black bean burger, and sweet potatoes. I'll add a dab of Omega 3 margarine to promote a creamy texture.*

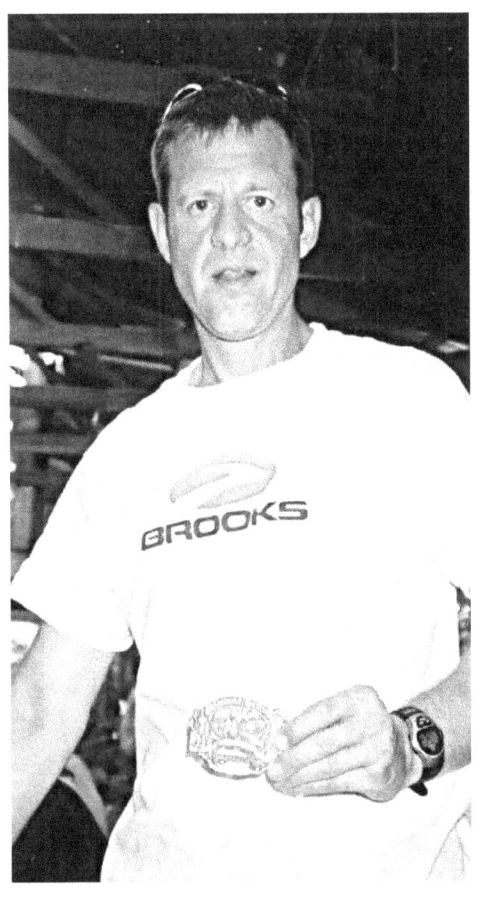

*A photo when I took one of my 100-mile finisher's buckles at the Mohican 100-mile race in Ohio. I have six finishes on the Mohican course. The 100-mile experience is a motivator in how I developed the Mind over Diet plan.*

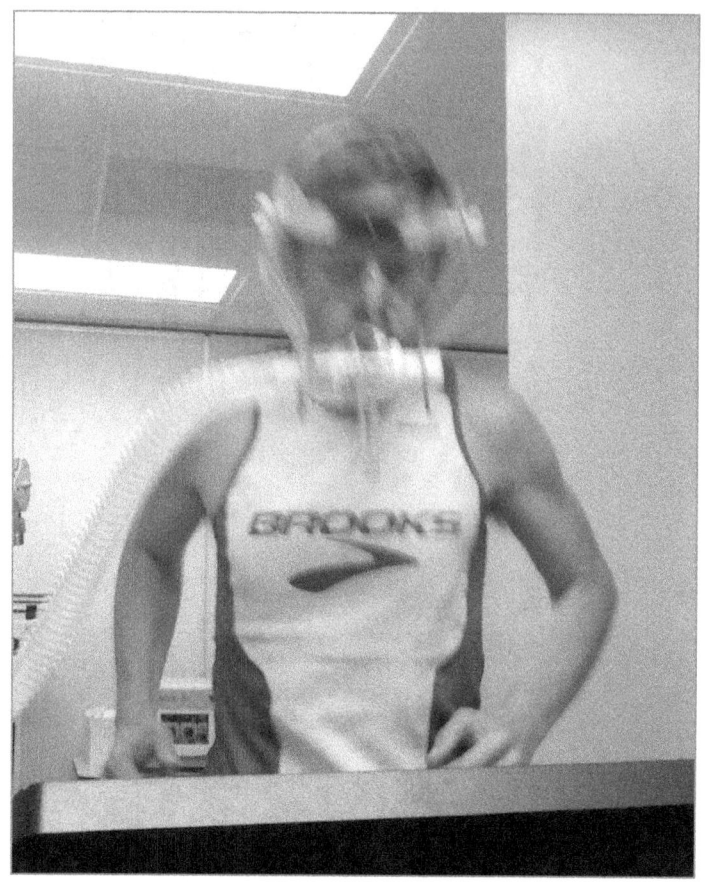

*This was my opportunity to gauge VO2 Max capacity. As an athlete, I'm nothing at all. On scale with ordinary individuals, I am exceptional. Mind over Diet keeps me excited and engaged in optimizing my body for the new adventures that are ahead.*

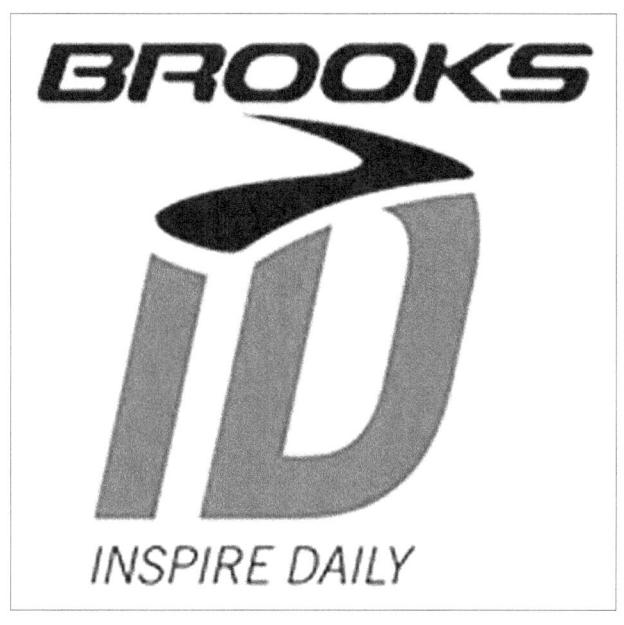

DISCLAIMER: I am a Brooks Sports promotional athlete for over 20 years. It's been a great journey and I appreciate the "Inspire Daily" mantra in both my academic and endurance sport activities.

# Daily Nutrition Breakdown

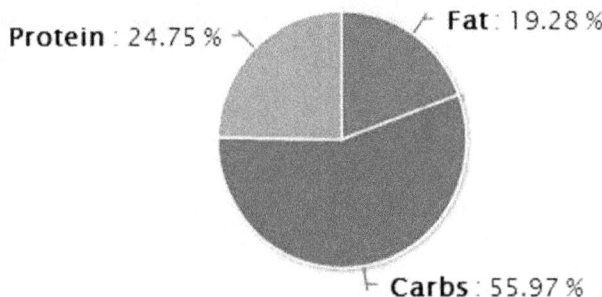

Protein : 24.75 %　　　　Fat : 19.28 %

Carbs : 55.97 %

Percentages based on your daily caloric intake

*Charting your food intake through one of the popular web-based or smart phone apps is essential. Here's how one of my days tracked for carbs, fats and protein. Based on your Mind over Diet analysis, how would this fit for your daily allocation?*

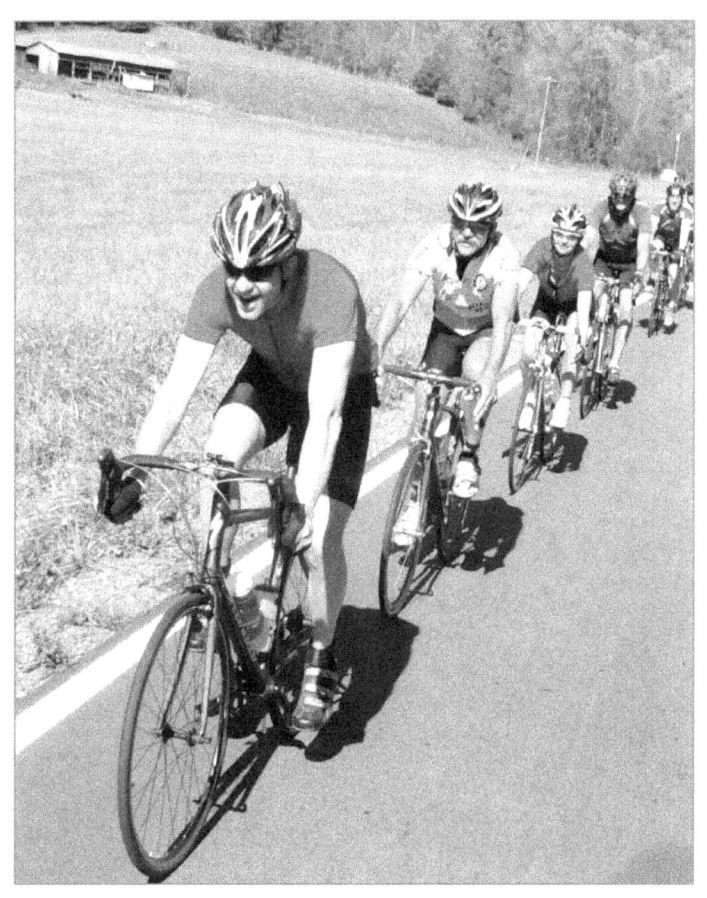

*The Mind over Diet fitness component is based on a wide variety of "always on" activities. You will self-negotiate the length and intensity of each fitness session to create a positive psychological schema.*

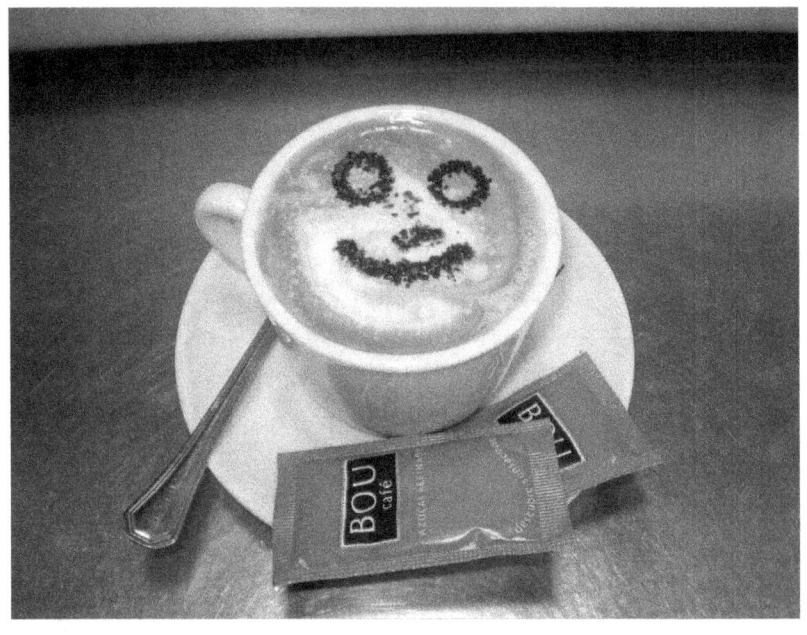

*A happy moment in the making: A fresh cappuccino served at a sidewalk café somewhere in Europe. Coffee is one of my guilty pleasures, in that it's low calorie, low fat and tremendously satisfying.*

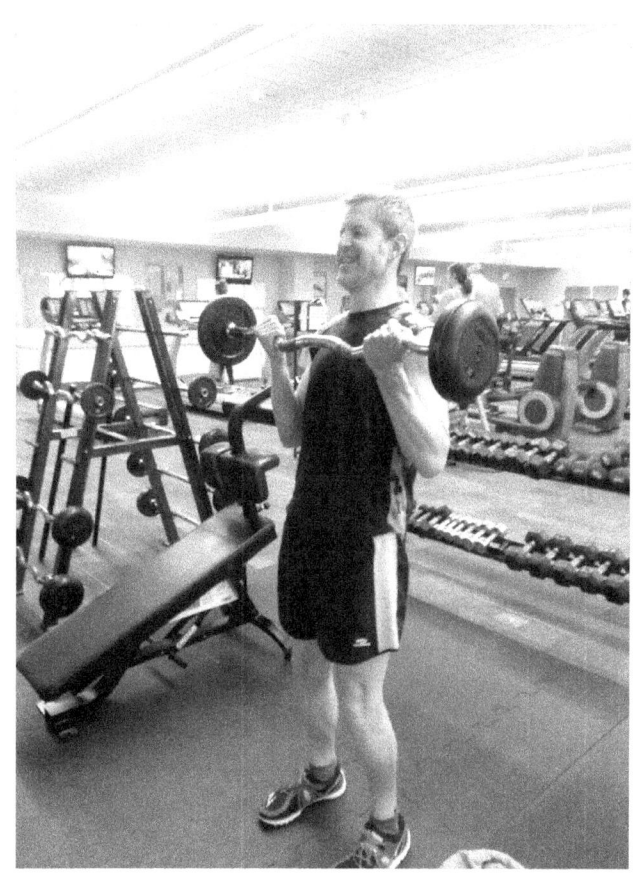

Consider strength training as a foundational piece in your Mind over Diet fitness plan. I like to start with 30 reps with this 30-pound barbell. It's not considered heavy. I'm more concerned with consistent movement.

My overuse tendencies went on for decades. Before Mind over Diet, I was engaged in what I though was mind over body. Just push harder, for longer, to bring my physical being into submission. I had been setting long term life goals that would deliver what I thought were necessary outcomes. Under that premise, massive exercise chunks were necessary every day.

I can recall one specific year when I ran a 50-mile race in April, a 50-mile race in May, and then a 100-mile race in June. Oh by the way, I threw 3-4 marathons into that mix and used them as training runs. How's that for a start to an athletic season? The sad part was, it was never enough and it was also about a fleeting validation.

On another occasion I entered a race in northern Michigan. It was a 50-mile and I attended with some of my best friends. One of my buddies was on my pace and we went back and forth throughout the event, seldom more than 25 yards apart. After one rather difficult woods section, my friend pulled ahead and then surged on the road section that followed. When I got out of the woods, he was gone. My friend beat me that day and I remained rather pouty afterwards. It wasn't so much that he beat me, but that I perceived I had beat myself, that I should have gone faster, performed better. My friend admonished, "Can't you ever be happy?"

I recall that painful experience in Mind over Diet to make a clear example of myself, in my own failures over the years, so that you can reflect and make sure that your fitness identity does not become a monster in your life. There is a place for exercise and possible affiliated events. You'll learn everything you need in this chapter to develop that component. But please understand your lust for social identity and the related psychology of training, fitness and results can be dangerous. Let's build our programs to assure that our fitness identity is working for us and that we aren't working as a slave to our fitness identity.

That's another self-disclosure for this discussion: I had over-prioritized my social identity through ultrarunning. When other parts of my life, business and personal, were not going well, I clung to the one area where I perceived I could force success. So in that era, I had to finish 100-mile races. It was a validation that (I thought) I couldn't live without.

I was also selfish with the exercise component in my life. Training can be time consuming. There was a specific day I can remember. I was in the garage, readying my bike and equipment for a long day on the road. A loved one told me "you have a very selfish sport." That day hangs in my mind as a lasting lesson of how exercise, training and related endurance sport is inherently a self-aggrandizing activity.

There are good outcomes, in how we care for our bodies and refresh our minds. However, it cannot become a bigger priority than our other responsibilities in life. It's important that as you make your own Mind over Diet plan, you balance changes in your life using consideration for those who you love, and in turn love you.

This book is a push-back against that form of thinking. For anyone who associates identity within sport, please step back and organize your schema to assure your social identity is multifaceted. We must strive to maintain several identities in our lives. I'd suggest we owe our identities to others, as well as ourselves. You might need a healthy identity as a parent, or civic club leader, or husband, wife or partner.

I realize that things seldom fall into place as we would have it. On most occasions, we shuffle the deck and push forward with the cards we are dealt. But throughout whatever surprises we find on our path, we must care for ourselves in a thoughtful and meaningful way. We must also care for others around us and much of that is a derivative of how we care for ourselves. If we're settled and can embrace our inner lives, the more we can love and show compassion to those around us.

For Mind over Diet practitioners, that means a logical process of self-discovery which is kind and gentle. It's never "all or nothing" regarding outcomes.

Consider that as you develop your Mind over Diet lifestyle, you can add a new social identity to your arsenal – that of encourager, advocate and cheerleader. I believe in the "pay it forward" approach to life and whenever possible, invest in others.

Several weeks ago, I received an email from an old friend. This individual reminded me that I was there when she first attempted a fitness plan, at a time she was sedentary and overweight. She recalled my encouraging nature and the fact I told her there was no shame in walk breaks intermixed with running. Fast forward several years and this person is now exceptionally fit and carries a positive, encouraging attitude of her own. She's such a success story that a major gym and fitness center features her images as part of its marketing and promotion materials.

My initial words, presented in a kind and inviting fashion, had a profound effect. You may start in the same place, tentative and unsure about your fitness future. But as I stated then and as I will underscore now, encouraging others is a potent psychological element. After you build your plan, consider helping others who have yet to engage the positive and active lifestyle you have attained. You can't put a price tag or value on friends or acquaintances who circle back to state you were the impetus in their Mind over Diet life conversion.

Now that we know that sharing encouragement is good, but that pursuing fitness can be a two-edged sword, where do we go next?

Think about the sport and exercise activities that make you find motivating. For example, I enjoy cycling and equipment related to that sport. It's fun to look at bikes and parts. It's also interesting to note that if a bike is light and strong, it isn't cheap. Or if it's low price (cheap) it won't be both light and strong. Alternately, if it's strong, it won't be light and cheap.

Our bodies, and bicycles, are not that dissimilar. I'll bring forward the "healthy, fit and light, pick two" scenario for your review and enjoyment. For on most any given day, you'll find yourself on top of two dimensions, but crashing and burning on the third. Let's play with it for a second.

Being healthy becomes a near impossibility for a master's age competitor. Injuries are nagging and sometimes heal slowly, if at all. I blew out my shoulder in a mountain biking accident and had an anaphylactic reaction to a wasp sting; two ER visits a month apart is not what I had in mind for that summer's undertakings. During some seasons of life, I am forced to fight through a flair-up of plantar fasciitis in my right foot, or my L-5/S-1 disc will touch the nerve and send me into pain management mode. What ailments are you fighting through? As we age, it's many times important to cope, not overcome.

"Light" comes and goes and can be elusive. There is no perfect world in endurance sport. Starting a race with all the stars lined up most often does not happen. I can recall a race where I was off a bit on light (had ballooned up to 173) and fit (had only completed two 10 mile runs in the past couple of months).

However, I was healthy. The bad disc in my back had offered me a reprieve, based in part on the fact my Mind over Diet fitness analysis had steered me away from the 70 mile running weeks that exacerbated it. So I've been in the gym every day and threw in a bit of mountain biking. When you're 56 and trying to stay relevant in endurance sport, it's not going to be perfect. I took what I had and went with it.

Setbacks ebb and tide but sometimes do not release you completely. I spoke with a rather famous ultrarunner who disclosed he has struggled with plantar fasciitis (foot pain) for the past three years. We may aspire to healthy, but on a 1 to 10 scale, many of us train and race at a 5 or 8.

Compounding the challenges related to injury, attaining "fit" is elusive. And, we need to aspire to something that is adaptable and achievable over the rest of our lives.

What's the vision for success in your personal fitness program? There may be a range to your goal setting. I'm 6 feet, 1 inch tall and can range from 153 to 180 pounds. Some of the elite ultrarunners are my height and hit the scales at 145 or 150. You may aspire to be lighter, which translates to faster, but it depends how engaged you become. Many times it comes down to a battle of the attitude - food or fit? At one point I was carved at 5% body fat and 160 pounds, then on another occasion 3% body fat and 153 pounds.

Please understand that big changes require a convergence of attitude, diet and fitness. For me, it's not unusual to run 10 miles in the morning then cycle for 2-3 hours (in the mountains) in the afternoon. Is that sustainable? Is it realistic as advice to others who want to build a Mind over Diet opportunity?

It wasn't long term. As each diet and fitness surge hit crescendo, work realities set in, my diet fell off, and injuries hit. So as "fit" increases, so does the risk for injuries. That will pull you down on the healthy dimension. No matter how you balance fit, light and healthy, the dimension of "happy" must also exist. It's a positive, all is well with the world mindset that is sporadic at times. The challenge is, how can we employ happy within all the possible contexts and outcomes?

Take away healthy or fit and watch the positive attitude drain out of your disposition. There's a verse in the bible that says we shouldn't build our faith on a sand foundation. I can't help but parallel that to how I built many of my former fitness peaks. I thought that big miles and a perfect diet were the rock solid cornerstones that would lead to happiness. It didn't work then, it won't work now. It becomes a pseudo life; I don't always like that about myself and work to build that foundation on a more diverse scale.

That's where the ongoing engagement of Mind over Diet must take place. We reach out and explore new information, new concepts and then self-negotiate our adapted next steps. After over 30 years of daily adherence to the endurance sport lifestyle, I can assure you that pursuing knowledge and implementing changes are a core component in long-term success.

On my most recent expedition back into an adapted food plan and workout routine, I had to delve into new information that freshened up my motivation. I stepped into the Paleo movement, not to disapprove or criticize, but rather to dig beneath the surface and understand the core premises that were attracting millions of advocates. Within that process, I noted the heavy emphasis on diet, with a lesser focus on exercise. Some of the top Paleo preachers were ripped, happy and only working out about 30 minutes a day.

I finally accepted that fact our diets should be the driver, seasoned with the spice of fitness. It wasn't about tearing my body to shreds through more and more workouts, then recklessly consuming uncontrolled portions of food. I needed to balance intake and output in a sensible way.

The chink in my armor was that of ignoring the consequences of unbridled eating. You may have heard an individual state, "I can eat anything I want, I'm a runner." Please know it's not true. On a good day, I could eat my way well past 10-mile runs.

The approach of sensible fitness coupled with nutritious eating is mandatory during the later stages of life. As the decades march by, it's impossible to sustain big miles, bit workouts, big racing spectacles. Our bodies just can't take the torque. We must transition to kinder, gentler versions of our former selves. That's a big schema piece for me and also a point of cognitive dissonance. I'm no longer known as racer or runner but instead author and enthusiast and encourager of others. I had to learn to take value out of the identity that is within my grasp, not an identity that has slipped away.

Our fitness component must bring value and a return on our investment, but it must not define us, or abuse us, or take us to that unhappy state. Instead we march forward, imperfect yet making sense of the world around us. I'm not completely healthy, not completely fit, and am working on being content. But despite it all I'm glad to be facing each day. Despite our shortcomings, we stay in the game and enjoy what we have to work with. The clay may be lumpy, but we craft it into an interesting work of art.

The years are slipping by and one unintended outcome is a decrease in prior performance, both running and on the bicycle. It started over a year ago and has continued into this season's club cycling sessions. I am quickly becoming the last rider in the pack, in some cases miles off the pace of other club participants. Call it social identity or my own self-inflicted stereotype of who I am on two wheels, but I find my lack of speed and endurance embarrassing and sometimes shameful.

When compared to others, I don't do well. My times are much slower, my heart range isn't as high as it used to be and I haven't won an age group award in many years. Being part of the cycling club is a big social identity piece. "Keeping up" was part of my social identity and was part of being accepted. Club members will wait for me at the turns, but being the guy pulling up the rear brings a deep melancholy that's hard to describe.

Several months ago I was on a cycling club ride, a 50-miler and a nice sunny day in the mountains of North Carolina. Early in the loop I realized that my best effort was not enough. I seemed to be a bit off song, but there's no excuses to be had in that. As the riding pack crested the next hill, they were gone. I was alone, and despondent, and carrying the shame of being the last rider.

On another occasion I "ran" a 50K in a forested area of North Carolina. It was a quaint little event, where I had a nice visit doing the miles with an old friend I have been running with for 25 years. The downside was my pace. I completed the course in a bit over 8 hours and came in second to last.

Ever finish a race at the tail end of the pack? It's not pretty. The race promoter seemed impatient and more than ready to shut down the finish line; there were two cars in the parking lot and the remaining post-race food consisted of a few lonely scones. The remnants of goodies left memories of those who enjoyed the post-race party, where many laughed and told race tales hours prior to my access to the food table.

I'd like to tell you it's all good, but it hurts. I'm getting slower each season, yet still want to be part of the sport. My ego gets in the way. I was never a winner, but for decades was a solid top 1/3 of the field runner. But that was then, this is now, and I'm bringing up the rear at most events.

Left to an unmanaged schema, one might spin into a funk. I have done that, but it's not acceptable. I may hit the wall and fall off the pace, but it's impossible to have every case study of life play out just as we intend. I may want to be a rock star, but on some days, I'm only a rock picker.

I wish there was a magic elixir that would restore the luster of our former performances. But when it's not possible we must push into an adaptive mode, accepting ourselves and our fitness and sport at a revised pace. Sometimes we try just as hard, but perform less. Fitness is about commitment and staying in a routine. One day truly doesn't matter (at least not physically), but my psyche was shouting that if I missed a workout, I'd come away feeling guilty and out of shape.

I seldom take a day off from exercise and continue to believe it's viable to sustain an every-day schedule. Giving your body a rest is important, but there are parameters to accomplish rest while pursuing a fitness session. Endurance sport may have extracted a toll, but I continue to enjoy the effort.

When I hit a really low point, which usually leads to me pouting while riding, I start to assess several important variables. That's a signal it's time to reset my compass and calibrate back to true north.

I am in the midst of a severe schema shift where I perceive myself as successful on many fronts, rather than a loser in a competitive sense. I remind myself that it's really not about me. I focus back on the model of agape love, which is to strive for caring about others over self. My performance on a bicycle pales in comparison to what sort of example I set or of how I relate to others who may be dealing with truly serious issues.

On one occasion I was in pout mode about my riding ability when I learned a friend of mine had just been informed his wife wanted a divorce. That was a Mind over Diet moment, in the sense I needed to absorb that information and reset my schema to put another's needs over my own.

I can remain in the sport and life I have loved for the past three decades, or I can get out. It's my choice. Most all of the guys and gals I ran and cycled with over the past 30 years have fallen off the routine and left the sport. I have decided that I will embrace the sport I love, albeit at a slower and more forgiving pace.

If you are last, or the least accomplished in a setting like the gym or yoga, it can be demoralizing. But it's not big or strong enough to define us. I may be last, but I'm getting great exercise at my own pace. It's up to me to determine what my athletic performance means to me, not what my performance means to others. I may be last, but it's not about me. Life is about how I can help and be an example to others.

We don't know what's in store for the future and we surely can't predict what our quest will become. I continue to have a passion for endurance sport and what it does in people's lives. I encourage others; that was the premise of

Mind over Diet. Emotion wells up inside me when I see individuals get strong on the inside through accomplishments in running and cycling. The revelation "I can do this!" resonates deep and a stronger human emerges.

There's another upside in finding identity in endurance sport. Over the three decades I've been part of the scene, I have been active in clubs and riding groups. Embracing the camaraderie and passion that bubbles up from a shared passion is infectious. I love to read Internet posts and emails about what rides are upcoming and what groups are coming together. But in that endearment I find a deep inner fear. If we slow down, will we lose our association with this cluster of friends? What will come of this group and the trials, tribulations and victories we encountered together?

So here I am, declawed, still dreaming of years past and former memories. That's not a bad thing, but I am packing some of that material into my archived schema folders and opening a few additional files entitled, "receptive to new ideas and interests and relationships."

When times seem bleak and my athletic prowess seems almost dead stop, I repeat the calming influence that comes when I repeat the mantra, "it's not about me." Life is about reaching out to others over self. If I'm off the back on club rides, that gives me a chance to interact with new riders coming into the sport. Encouraging others creates an alternative payback. I can no longer carry the speed I once was capable of, but I can help others embrace their riding experience.

With a good understanding of how our minds must be engineered to embrace a new, gentle yet persistent mindset, let's delve into how your plan will create a strong return on fitness investment.

**Research a social media photo sharing site and run a search for "female fitness" or "male fitness."**

The images you access will be astounding and possibly intimidating. A huge challenge and potential obstacle to Mind over Diet fitness development is the vision we create for ourselves, based on an unrealistic self-assessment, or based on the achievements of others in the media or in our lives.

Some individuals in the fitness coaching arena are other-worldly. There's a new catch phrase "strong is the new sexy" and that surely plays out in the modern world of fitness. The cut, toned, shredded and ripped specimens portrayed in gym settings seem to have little to do with the world we'll create using the Mind over Diet philosophy. It's good to set goals but remain cautious about your intentions. Be deliberate and employ your tactics slowly and methodically. Quick achievements and shortcut body building programs seldom last after the goal is achieved, if they are achieved at all.

We've all been inundated with advertorial shows on TV; the premise of most is that with very little effort, you can drop massive pounds and look like a ripped free-weight model. Many programs are bogus, but some do seem to produce results. These extended DVD packages with support materials run in the hundreds of dollars. Several brands are available and combine cardio, weight resistance and stretching.

There are aerobic and strength programs that profess 10 minutes a day, 25 minutes a day, or some are 90 minutes a day. Product users profess results and report solid advancements, many times over a 60 or 90 day period.

If you exercise at extreme levels, you'll be dropping dozens of pounds in no time, correct? I feel a dull thud hit my stomach when I see these propositions for success. Every form of fitness has some benefit, but few, if any, will achieve the "fitness male" or "fitness female" outcome without a strict and regimented food plan.

**Use your favorite Internet search engine to explore the calories expended with various forms of exercise.**

If we developed a total anaerobic motion for 10 minutes, how many calories might that burn? Check your own sources, but I'd suggest a maximum output for that short duration might be 300 calories.

Calories related to both food and exercise is not an exact science. But it is a great measuring tool for advancement with fat loss and fitness. Think again about that hard, 10-minute workout. If we performed that effort seven days a week, we'd be looking at a 2100 calorie fitness effort.

Now let's match that calories expenditure against a couple of eating decisions. A popular chocolate and caramel candy bar comes in at 380 calories. So, your weekly exercise equals a little over 5.5 candy bars. Here's another comparison: A medium chocolate shake from a fast food restaurant is approximately 580 calories. So if you're into a few shakes each week, you can trade your exercise plan for 3.6 of these thick treats.

It all has to work together. We'll develop a refreshed positioning of the mind, the right foods, and a consistent fitness plan. Let's do some simple math. If you're attempting to become the ultimate specimen and you're expecting to do that through the 10 minute intensity plan each day, here's where you might engage the calorie count.

It's a tough parameter, but let's say you can exist on 1500 calorie a day diet. That's almost starvation territory, but with exceptional discipline, it's possible. Living on 1500 a day is brutal, I've been there. Let's say we were eating 2500 a day so now we carved out 1000. Under this scenario, we would accomplish:

- Exercise plan burns 2100 calories per week
- Reduction of 7000 calories per week through reduced food intake
- Calorie advantage minus 4900 per week equals approximately 1.5 pound loss per week

That's six pounds a month, 18 pounds over 90 days. Not a bad program, but much of the advantage comes through food reduction, not the 10 minute exercise burn. The problem for me is that 99% of the pitch is about the workout plan, not the diet. I realize purchasing decisions are based on outcome with the least effort expended. A consumer clutches to the possibility of flailing around for 10 minutes a day and looking shrink-wrapped.

Another popular movement also advocates a light exercise routine. The Paleo diet lifestyle intrigues me. It's weight bearing and minimal. Many of the big name Paleo proponents advocate a short duration of exercise a day, usually a brief cardio warm-up and then variations of body strength resistance.

Some Paleo advocates believe calories don't count, rather that the content of the calories matter most. A recent podcast stated that athletes, in some cases women, were "skinny fat" through a non-Paleo diet and in their opinion, excessive exercise. Thin on the outside, fat on the inside.

It's at this juncture nutrition and sport enthusiasts need to reach a decision point: I believe you're either purpose training, or vanity training. Much of the Paleo world is about being ripped, or in its latest configuration, shredded. Men are often shirtless to expose sets of ab muscles.

I must say that over the snowy winter months, you might find me working the circuit training machines, doing a bit of vanity training myself. Others, let's say those who intend on completing a 13.1 or 26.2 mile running event, might opt for purpose training. When I am prepping for a distance running event, I complete runs of 10 miles or more on many occasions. Some runs are in excessive heat and on occasion I can feel the sometimes painful yet promising burn in my stomach. It's indicative of fat cells being cooked at a rapid pace.

We must build our bodies to perform for the outcome we desire. Fifteen minutes of jumping jacks isn't going to get me to the top of a mountain on our next club cycling ride. Our personal choices are what build the Mind over Diet plan. We determine the level of aerobic fitness necessary as part of our personal finish line.

I'm not adhering to either vanity training or purpose training, but I do want to promote the debate. What makes you motivated? At present, I'll adhere to maintenance for winter mixed with some vanity goals. But I don't plan on being "skinny fat" anytime soon.

I want to make another important point: Do not launch a fitness plan that creates a sure opportunity for you to fail. Your primary goal is to understand the timeline for your fitness lifestyle is "forever." It's an easy and methodical engagement, with small digestible adaptations when needed.

For most, it won't be a jump around 30 minutes a day DVD workout, or high-intensity interval training (HIIT). If you haven't yet come across HIIT, you will. It's all the rage now, suggesting that less, in very hard and high doses, plays out as more.

I'm not suggesting that HIIT isn't beneficial, but I am saying it hurts and is unpleasant and for most, won't be a motivator to continue on future days. What matters most is how you engage your Mind over Diet research, then determine an action plan. You are the author and it's your personal road map. You'll self-negotiate what you will do, to what intensity, and when you will do it.

That's one big selling point for Mind over Diet. It presents the best fitness plan of all time.

When you take the proper steps to educate yourself, reorder your schema, and reset your social identity, you will have ownership of a fitness scenario that defensible. Out of thousands of fitness and exercise plans, you will have created the one superior program, which stands clearly over the competition in both definition and ROI.

Here's what the long view has allowed me to understand: The best fitness program ever created is the one you stay engaged in over a long period of time.

Most of those who started in endurance sport with me in the mid 1980's are long gone. When their speed lessened and age group wins were no long possible, they faded away. Some individuals "bucket list" endurance sport, finish a couple of high profile events, then exit. Countless others have come into, and then out of, a fitness lifestyle over the decades. When you identify those who keep engaging year after year, it's a low percentile.

I'm here to advocate that if you are exercising, find that place you can maintain. If you're not, let me help you gain the foothold needed to bring a fitness component into your life, for the long haul.

First, set a minimum amount of time you will invest every day. For starters 15 minutes might work, or maybe 30 minutes is an optimal goal. Fill that time with whatever is sustainable. At first it may be stretching, an easy morning walk, or a smooth swim. Make it as easy as necessary, but don't miss the commitment. You are building the plan on your own terms. At one point I had a 3.5 year streak going where I didn't miss a day of running. My minimum was a 30 minute jog. I can remember several evenings, out at 11:30 pm, getting it done to keep the streak alive.

After you have determined your minimum fitness duration per day, continue to engage your daily activity based on time, rather than distance, reps or intensity. Too often, we become slaves to statistics where it's essential to hit a certain distance, at a certain speed. Or we must complete a certain number of repetitions and a certain number of sets in the gym.

Throw that mindset in the dirty towel bin. Instead, be gentle with yourself. It's a life commitment. As we age, we slow, so hitting the "marks" may no longer be possible. Set your mind on the time allotted each day, then fill it. You may have intended to jog, but if you're tired, take a slow spin on your bike or go to a yoga class. You are successful because you engaged the minimum time commitment.

In contrast, have you ever observed someone attempting to adhere to a strict, prefabricated training program? Recently, the 13.1 mile half marathon is all the rage and of course marketers have come quickly to bring 13.1 nutrition plans, training programs and social identity monikers. Have you seen the 13.1 decal on cars?

Proponents of these plans many times miss daily prescribed workouts and their schemas shift. They psychologically defeat themselves, believing they cannot complete the race because the detailed training plan is not complete. Or, the rigors of maintaining a difficult, unpleasant workout day after day defeats the runner's will to continue.

In the Mind over Diet fitness plan, we are "always on." This may be controversial, but I don't believe in skipping exercise days. It's a psychological advantage. As mentioned, many times individuals miss one session and in turn break momentum. Then it's easier to miss the second consecutive day of training and before long, good bye fitness and hello blubber tummy.

Of course, there are extenuating circumstances. I may have international travel days, but even then I'm walking 1-2 miles in the airports. Manage the effort in each session, but don't miss altogether. I may take an "off" day and instead ride my commuter bike on errands. It's easy and fun and integrated into my normal activities. The exercise regime is sustained.

Build slowly and always maintain. As the days tick by and you've held your commitment to the 30 minute (or whatever time you choose) sessions, you will become stronger in mind and body. Confidence will come into the equation. When you are ready, incrementally alter your workouts. Maybe it's a few sit ups, or a short burst of speed at the end of your walk. It's your plan, your outcome, and there are no rules with the exception of one, to keep the streak alive.

Months may pass and you'll set a new self-agreement; your sessions are stepping up to 60 minutes a day, with a 30 minute minimum. Or, you may want to stay on 30 minutes forever. Just remember, the plan that works is the one you keep in motion over time.

Now that you have a base understanding of how the greatest fitness plan of all time is developed, what are the next steps? There are tens of thousands of individuals slouched on the couch, wishing there were a way to get back into the fitness game. There is a sure way and we're going to unpack it in the next few pages. There are several different forms of fitness activities you may wish to explore.

**For each of the italicized headings that follow, use your favorite search engine to research the fitness activities. Each has potential as you build your personal Mind over Diet fitness protocol.**

*Strength training*

Several months ago, I heard a news report that changed the way I approached my fitness planning. The article stated that one of the major detractors of quality of life, later in life, is related to how feeble you become.

What's feeble? There are several dictionary definitions, but in essence becoming feeble entails a declining strength factor, overall weakness, a related reduction in the power of the mind, which leads to an overall reduction in quality of life.

The opposite of weak, is strong. As we age, strength training is optimally important for performance. Being old and wispy shouldn't figure into my future plans, or yours. I have dabbled in strength training in prior decades, but always put it on the back burner because I was chasing a maximum calorie burn every day – usually because I needed to offset overeating or poor eating habits.

There are many approaches to strength training. Much of the media imaging is centered on males and females who have amassed huge bodies and bulking muscles, gained through supplements and hours in the gym each day. Other sources have suggested that simple body weight exercise, done intensely in short duration, will actually deliver as much benefit in the long run.

Many fitness programs are marketed to highlight more mass, bigger muscles, a chiseled abdominal section, and massive arms. To gain the results purported, most strength training recommendations will take you "to exhaustion." When you are designing the strength portion of your Mind over Diet fitness plan, consider if your activities will entice and motivate, day after day. Whenever I go to exhaustion, it's most always a bad experience. Exhaustion brings pain and pain triggers negative schema files. Soon after, it may prompt a shutdown of that activity.

"No pain, no gain" may not be appropriate for you. I'm not advocating that hard work is bad, rather that you need to self-negotiate the pain threshold. Easy does it, lean in slowly, make short incremental changes. You're designing a long-term, always-on fitness scenario and you don't need to rush into the results. If you start a new strategy that reduces other fitness activity and invest in a new strength plan, implement the change over a substantial period of time. Use slow methodical motions. Remember that we're into the plan for the long haul and aren't looking for a quick fix or fast results.

Strength training does not have to entail a gym, expensive equipment, or the latest in home exercise equipment. A really appealing approach to strength training can be no equipment at all. There's a movement underway to embrace old-fashioned body weight exercises. Push-ups, squats, sit-ups, and other weight bearing variations can be used quite effectively. For example, I have use yoga poses to engage core muscles and have seen a noticeable increase in toning and strength. Approach your strength training protocol with the Mind over Diet system response, reading and listening to a wide variety of sources in order to become better educated about how to proceed. There are smart phone or tablet apps that coach you through a timed body weight exercise routine. Strength gain can be simple and done anywhere with this option. A fun option is to move your strength show outdoors, incorporating an exercise ball into crunches and pushups.

There are other gym-originated workouts. I like to use circuit training equipment, where you put a pin in a stack of weights to set your desire weight resistance, then push, pull or dip on that specific machine. Explore the various strength training approaches, as it regards the number of repetitions and the number of sets (grouped repetitions).

Consider slow, easy, methodical lifts. I go 15 repetitions, rest, and then do another 15 repetitions. It's an easy burn in my limbs and it gives me a toned defined look. A while back I thought about increasing the weight load but then decided against it. What I am currently doing is appealing and has me coming back for more. The nuance of strength training can become a moving target. We can embrace each new dimension and develop hybrid applications. Let's be good to ourselves and set goals that are gentle on the mind and soul, and are realistic to an age-appropriate model.

Would you try to disassemble a working plan that is attractive? There's always room for more, but it has to be tested to assure the challenge can be accommodated by your "always on" fitness routine. If it's not fun, or if it hurts too much, your schema will start planting negative files in your brain. If workouts are unpleasant, you will start to subliminally translate a formula that states "workouts do not equal fun." It's imperative that you challenge yourself and on some occasions reach for more, but not to the point you disconnect from the desire to engage on a daily basis.

Strength training delivers a substantial return on investment. When done properly and with realistic goals, weight bearing exercise will strengthen joints and bones and also make you more resilient. Have a sore back or a bad disc? Strength training will assist with building the core muscles, which will help to support the back and vertebrae.

And, strength training enhances the mind. Remember the naked test we discussed at the beginning of this book? You can invest 10-12 weeks in strength training, then "retest" in front of the mirror. Wow. That's the new you. Your body tightens; the muscles gain definition and form to sculpture your physique. Visual prompts sink deep into the psyche. You are strong, you are sleek and you have done it your way, all the way.

*Heart rate*

I was glancing at a chart in my university's recreation center. It was posted to educate patrons on heart rate zone training. Your heart rate is a useful measurement related to level of effort and is calibrated by the number of beats your heart produces each minute (beats per minute, or "bpm").

A common approach to determining your heart rate range starts by subtracting your age from 220; that's your max heart rate. Then take 60% of that amount for low range, 80% for high range, and you'll have the fat burn/training zone. Using myself as an example, it looks like this:

- 220-57 (years old) = 163 beats per minute
- 163 bpm x 60% = 98 bpm low range
- 163 bpm x 80% = 130 bpm high range

Other programs suggest a much lower range of effort that puts my bpm between 113 and 123 bpm. What's most important is that you start by benchmarking your resting heart rate and your exercising heart rate. Then, apply your starter rates to future efforts in Mind over Diet activity. In a perfect world, your resting rate should decrease, while your ability to increase exercise at a higher bpm should become more comfortable over time.

You can attain your heart rate by placing your index finger on the vein in your neck, or on your wrist, and count the number of beats for 10 seconds. Multiply that by six for a bpm reading. Or, there are many heart rate monitors on the market. Most operate through the use of a chest strap that reads your heartbeat directly. Also, some of the aerobic machines at the gym incorporate a pulse meter into hand positioning. Just this morning I did 60 minutes on a strider machine and observed my pulse as I exercised.

The theory for most heart rate training plans is that it's good to work hard so that you elevate your heart rate, adapt to higher bpm's, and perform at a faster pace. Pump the heart faster and faster and pretty soon you'll be hoisting the trophy at Boston or wearing the yellow jersey at a tour stage. Is that solid advice, or silly input?

As a Mind over Diet proponent it's my opinion that less bpm's is better. Some of the top ultrarunners in the USA can successfully complete 50-mile events while their heart rate hovers around the 100 bpm mark. Solid, methodical training brings our bodies into an efficient state of being. You may not be winning the race, but performing at a heart rate that isn't pinging off the rev limiter is much more enjoyable over long periods of time.

Back in 1993, I finished a 50-mile event in while not letting my heart rate top 130. I was dealing with health problems (coming off Guillain-Barre). Fast forward to present and I'm still competing in a low bpm range. My resting pulse is in the low 40's, I train at 100-130 and max at 139.

I usually hit max heart rate while doing the big climbs in our cycling routes. Sometimes I wish I had more – some of the riders who are my age continue to push a max of 170-180 bpm. But I am settled and satisfied with the Mind over Diet plan, as I created it, and will exist within those boundaries. Working to gain an additional 40 bpm's per minute might increase performance, but the effort and pain to get there would not be conducive to long term sustainability.

I'm not a world beater, but how many master competitor athletes are? If you're attempting to finish races and have fun, stay relaxed and see how far you can go with your pulse in low gear. Guess what? When your pulse is low you hurt less and smile more. Lower pulse equals a longer distributed effort. When I'm on my feet for 5-7 hours in a 50K, I'm not looking for 60 or 80 percent of my max; I'm looking for easy footfalls, relaxed breathing, and my engine at idle.

There are advocates who will encourage you to jack up your heart rate, while others will state that staying in a lower zone will bring you to a higher efficiency and better performance. It's best to investigate and take ownership of how you want to address heart rate, or if you wish to address it at all. You are in command, it's your call. Take a closer look and determine where you're headed and how you want to get there.

*Walking/jogging/running*

I recently made another attempt at finishing a 100-mile ultramarathon event. This race uses a multiple loop course and it's round and round, again and again, all day long and into the night. The winner brought it home in just less than 16 hours, while the female champion was only a few minutes back.

Bottom line, I ran an exceptional race by my standard. I kept the pulse rate low and interspersed walking with slow jogging. Most of my miles were in in the 12-15 minute range. Things were going well and I was able to complete 50-miles in 12 hours, 30 minutes. However, my feet went south and deteriorated. I made a smart decision and dropped out at 62 miles.

I haven't finished a 100-miler in some time. Much of it is about the way my schema processes decisions and I also experienced a shift in social identity. In 100-mile races, the prize for finishing is a belt buckle. At prior races, I took a finish but was crippled, needed medical attention, and could not walk for 10 days. My old schema screamed, "You must finish, you will only be validated by the finish."

When things weren't going well in my life, punching the 100-mile card was imperative to my social identity. Now, a softer, kinder personality has emerged. I'm an academic, a researcher, and one who chooses to model the Mind over Diet plan for others. I'm OK with my effort, however the day unfolds. I race less, with more focus on the fitness component.

If you're going to be a new entrant into the walking, jogging or running fitness world, foot care may be a paramount issue. Some of you will be able to wear inexpensive cotton socks and stay on your feet all day with no issues. Many runners cross the finish line at 100-mile race, giggle, and throw on some flip flops.

I'm not that person. Of my eight (8) 100-mile finishes I only made it through once without blasted, destroyed feet. It's a terrible thing and I strive to find a solution. I'm convinced that regarding blisters, you only get one shot.

You choose a shoe/sock/tape/lube/powder set up and go with it. If hot spots and then blisters emerge, you have to live with it or stop. I have never achieved improvement by messing with my feet during a race. I doctored my feet during several ultradistance events and it was a progression of increasing pain.

There are many modern choices in socks. Some products offer a double layer of fabric that is purported to diminish friction. Other fit like a glove with separate toe sleeves. Patches and dressings are available that are skin-like in texture and act as a second layer of skin. Books, web sites and blogs devoted to foot care. Hiking on uneven surfaces can exacerbate foot friction. Based on your own intentions with running or walking, you may need to address foot maladies.

Shoes are personal preference. We have encountered the barefoot and minimalist running craze. The minimalist movement said "less is better" and that is was more natural to run as the human body was designed. It's come to the best of both worlds. We now understand that low heel drop shoes make sense, but removing cushioning may be detrimental to most recreational runners.

I'd suggest you examine newer models of shoes that combine low heel drop and ample cushioning and stability.

Use your Mind over Diet research plan to explore and learn more. In the end, get a shoe that fits well. It doesn't matter what the latest marketing initiative purports. As the old saying goes, "If the shoe fits, wear it." And I'll an addendum that states, "If the shoe doesn't fit, don't run in it!"

As we work towards longevity and rewarding experiences, consider that there is a progression in foot-propelled exercise, from an easy walk, to a shuffling jog, to a slow run. More isn't better when you're doing daily exercise. And, it's not only pace that matters, it's how you carry your body while engaging in running.

I produced a video entitled *Most Efficient Running Technique* and if you're interested, you can find in on the Internet. I propose an easy, methodical pace where we visualize our feet turning over in a "tank track" motion. The foot motion is illustrated through an elliptical arc while keeping the turnover close to the ground. Feet low to the ground land more gently and produce less impact.

When running, it's possible to visualize a string that runs through the core of your body and out the top of your head. Imagine that someone above is pulling that string taut. Can you envision the tall, erect body form? Remember that the spine must carry our weight as we propel forward. I like to believe that my erect stance and easy foot strike best supports my somewhat fragile vertebra and instills prolonged health.

Adhering to the Mind over Diet personal planning model can be helpful to others. I have a friend who was attempting to embrace an exercise plan. She wanted to begin the journey to weight loss and improved health. We discussed running and I told her it didn't have to be full effort from the start. I suggested periods of walking that were interspersed with short, easy spurts of jogging.

Several years passed. Then I heard from my friend. Utilizing the easy-entry approach, she developed a plan that allowed her to "win" every day. She wasn't discouraged by someone forcing her to believe that faster and harder was a necessity. Rather, she leaned in slow and easy.

This individual has sustained the effort, interspersing with gym, weights, Pilates and yoga. I'm proud to report my friend is now a featured athlete in the marketing material at her gym. She's refreshed, rejuvenated and recharged, full of positive energy with a positive schema and healthy social identity. If there's a lesson here for us all, it's that a slow building process is important when you're building the effort and need to succeed.

I hope that you will consider a mix of walking and running as you build you Mind over Diet vision for fitness. I have run in points all across the globe and it's been a great activity and character-builder. Running is also an excellent social mixing opportunity. Check the Internet for local running clubs. There are also web sites that congregate people based on interests; I have used these sites to connect with diversified local runners in many international cities.

Running is also one of the most efficient calorie expenditure undertakings you can muster. Bust out the door, jog for 60 minutes at 11.5 minute miles, and extract somewhere around 830 calories from your body.

If you choose to walk or run in an outdoor environment, you may encounter hot and humid weather. Be aware of your hydration needs. This is once again an area where you need to become informed about what is best for your efforts. Some marketers will promote specific drinks, powders and devices designed to carry fluids.

I take a minimalist approach. When in race events, most ultra runs offer fluid stations every several miles. I usually choose a simple hand-held water bottle with retainer strap. However, quite a few others opt for a max load model. New racing packs are game changers – some fit like vests and mount dual water bottles at the chest, rather than around the waist.

When you're on your feet, walking or running at any speed, there is the element of the mind. It's how we engage, or disengage, that can set the psyche as the miles roll by. Consider if you would like to associate or disassociate with your running experience. I used to adhere to disassociating while running, loading my personal listening device with podcasts and digital books. There is a new option in the age of social media; some choose to run while texting on smart phones or checking real-time streaming results from the event. Others walk and jog in packs, talking about diverse life issues.

On other occasions, associating with the run and the experience seems right. During a recent 100-mile run, I started to enjoy the silence, the sound of my foot strike, coupled with deep personal thoughts about my place in the world.

When you do walk or run, take advantage of the one of the biggest motivators available to Mind over Diet athletes and smile. I have learned to paint a big smile on my face and leave it there. During a recent running event, there were two out and back spurs on the course, which allowed interaction with oncoming traffic. My smile bred friendship. I noted that as the laps went by, more folks started engaging me. Also, a smile bleeds into your soul. After 40 or 50 miles, you need to deeply embrace the good and positive within the experience.

I hope this section will prime your interest in building your own walking and jogging initiatives. It's possible the running bug will bite and you'll find enjoyment in the activity. Running can present an enjoyable personal challenge. Some might consider watching spectator sport, but in running, you can become an active participant in the sport.

*Bicycling*

Bicycling is a wonderful opportunity to combine machinery and the human body into an efficient, sensory experience. I have been cycling in many forms for the past 30 years and would like to share some of the opportunities that exist.

I'm tailoring this portion of the book to beginner level riders (please bear with me if you are an advanced wheeler). Consider the various forms of modern cycling. There are road bikes, "fat" bikes, mountain bikes (downhill and cross country), cyclocross bikes, commuter bikes, touring bikes and hybrid bikes. Frames for these machines are formed from aluminum, carbon fiber, steel or titanium. Most of these bikes feature multiple gear options that allow you to adjust the level of effort as you ride on hills, flats or downhill. Also common to off road bicycles is the integration of shock absorbers, most commonly in the fork (front) assembly but many times also in the rear portion of the frame, which allows the rear wheel to better absorb impact.

Use your Mind over Diet exploration skills and search several Internet sites that depict how bikes are ridden and what communities they engage. I'm sorry to report that some cyclists are friendlier than others. I don't know where it started but a level of arrogance has been inbred into road cycling. Why be elitist? Maybe it comes from the skin tight "kits" and $6000 machines these riders choose to ride.

There is no need for that attitude. Mind over Diet proponents are warm and inviting to all riders at all levels. We live to encourage others. When we strive to encourage cyclists and enhance their positive experience it can present a personal schema builder and social identity enhancement.

Here is a quick overview of how you might incorporate cycling into your aerobic planning. First, consider the type of riding you would like to attempt and then examine the risk associated with that form of cycling. For instance, if you live in a high traffic area, road riding might entail some stressful moments as you share the road with motorists. Mountain biking can lead to rather precarious trails and if you are not skilled in riding technical terrain, it's possible to take a trip over the handlebars.

If you have no prior cycling experience, I would suggest an entry level road bike. It's the most versatile; you can use it for commuting, for greenway and rails-to-trails exploring, and as an entry point to local cycling clubs and events. Many times, there are good values in used equipment. Your local bike shop may have bikes that have been traded in, or there are other local buy-and-sell sites on the Internet. I enjoy shopping for used bikes and consider it a hobby. Two of my current bikes were purchased used. They were almost new and I was able to purchase them at about half of retail cost.

Riding a bike requires balance, multitasking (hands, eyes and feet) and the ability to shift from sitting standing riding positions. If possible, find a veteran cyclist who can assist in your learning curve. If you're a veteran cyclist and you're reading this book, become a mentor to others who need encouragement and a helping hand.

In addition to the bikes, there are equipment considerations. A high quality helmet is a must and most will opt for special cycling shoes that allow your foot to "lock" into the pedal. This allows for a more powerful pedal spin and better riding technique. There are also apparel options, such as padded cycling shorts (yes, please!) and riding tops that offer rear pouches for carrying gear and food.

Be sure to locate local bike clubs. Reach out and attend a ride or meeting. Learn what the club is about and the opportunities available. Larger communities many times offer a wider dispersion of riding interests and pace. For example, I am quite active with a subset of our local club. Some faster subgroups are all about the pace, while our group adheres to relaxed attitude and focus on social interaction.

I must say I'm directionally challenged and love my club ride leaders. They take us through the back roads and valleys in our region and I never have to worry about getting lost. I simply follow the pack and enjoy the journey.

Other members in our club are active in our new mountain bike park. I tried the loop there and had a terrible crash. After my shoulder healed I opted out of that terrain and instead, ride mountain bikes solo in another more forgiving riding area. Cycling requires that we adapt to our own motivations and abilities.

If you would like to use cycling as a fitness component in your Mind over Diet plan, it can either be recreational or something completely different. Getting faster and becoming elite requires a committed cycling fitness plan and numerous rides with a competitive cluster of athletes.

Here's a scenario that I use. First, there on season versus off season cycling efforts. In the winter months, we enjoy sporadic rides "off the mountain" when the weather window allows. In the warmer months (and when there is more daylight) it's not unusual to do a long 50-60 mile ride Saturday, then three or more weeknight rides of 30-40 miles each. And on Sundays, I head to a mountain bike park after church and do a three hour solo ride. There are other instances where I'll use my commuter bike (an old converted mountain bike with panniers) for easy greenway spins or to run errands.

Depending on the group, the effort can be from easy to quite strenuous. Some days I want an easy ride while on others, I'll want to test my stamina against others in the riding group. There's something magical about sharing a big effort with friends. I sometimes joke, "I am a legend in my own mind!" as I push a climb and imagine what mountain stage riders must experience in the world cycling races.

One of the essentials for Mind over Diet cyclists is awareness. It's a mindfulness of who is around you, both motorists and other cyclists. It's scanning the road ahead and possible danger points. It's being conscious of your riding partners and their speed.

Beware of "pace lines." Pacing is a cycling term that indicates riders are in formation, in a long line, each riding 1-2 feet behind the rear wheel of the rider in front of them. This is called drafting; when you ride in the slipstream of air created by the rider in front of you, the effort you need to expend may be reduced by as much as 25 percent. Drafting does help but it can also be dangerous. It only takes one mistake and several riders can go down in an instant.

If you are new to a group or club ride, stay off pace lines until you are confident in your own ability and you also know the capability of the other riders in the line. Sometimes you may fall back from the group. Enjoy the ride and don't engage negative thoughts. At other times your riding partners may fall behind. It's best to regroup at turns and assure that everyone rested and ready to continue.

Bicycling is a wonderful consideration for your fitness routine. It continues to attract and motivate me year after year. The dual components of fitness versus equipment keep me going. When my body is optimized I can make the bike "sing" on the pavement. There's something magical about the hum of the tires and the chain spinning across the gears.

I'm not the cyclist I once was, based on overall performance. But when I view my cycling experience through a different lens I can identify camaraderie and wonderful social and outdoor experience. I hope that you can find the same reward where bicycling makes you fruitful, fulfilled and anticipating the next ride.

*Swimming*

If you want a gentle, graceful activity that takes the load off your legs and works alternative muscles, consider heading to the pool for regular swimming sessions. I have been swimming since my triathlon days and was never highly accomplished, but nonetheless came to appreciate the sport as a gentle form of exercise rather than a performance outcome.

There are great Internet sources for swimming videos that demonstrate nuance in the swim stroke (arms) and kick (legs). The most common swimming form is freestyle, which is forward motion face down in the water, using an overhead arm style and leg kicking for propulsion.

You'll also explore breathing techniques, which are set to timing of the strokes. As a beginner, you may want to twist your face out of the water for a breath on each stroke; as one arm enters the water your head is turned to the opposite side for a quick gulp of air. Once you get more experienced and relaxed in the water, you may need to breathe less. I'm not fast, but efficient. Over time, I have learned to take a breath every four to six strokes.

My swim workouts are one hour in length with no set distance parameters. I swim slow and easy, working to get a good "catch" with my hand as my arm enters the water and extends out front of my body. For the first 30 minutes, I use a foam float that fits between my legs. In this fashion, my body is aligned in the water but I can forgo the use of my legs and isolate my arm stroke. For the second half of the workout, I switch to hand paddles and foot flippers. This equipment gives a much greater "bite" in the water and propels your body forward with increased speed.

Consider how swimming might work for your personal Mind over Diet workout commitment. If you have self-negotiated a 30 minute a day exercise session, break down your swim workout within that time frame. It's possible to do 15 minutes freestyle with a leg float, then the final 15 minutes engaging the legs. Mix and match different elements to spice up your swim routine.

A key aspect of your swimming experience is related to aquatic eyewear. There are a variety of goggles on the market, some so tiny they fit inside the eye socket, while others are more scuba-like in design, seal around the eye area, and offer a panoramic view. There are also options for the shade of the lenses, from clear all the way to dark mirrored and reflective lenses. I used to swim in a 50 meter outdoor pool and opted for smaller goggles with blue tinted lenses. Now, when my swimming is indoors in a 25 meter pool, I opt for clear lenses and large format goggles.

I have a love and hate relationship with the pool and that's mostly due to my busy mind. Swimming is a cocoon-like activity with little interaction or input for the brain. I can concentrate on my arm stroke and kick, but even with that level of engagement, 60 minutes seems like a long time. I have purchased a waterproof sleeve and aqua ear buds for my personal listening device. On some occasions

I'll go through the bother of hooking it up so I can listen to a podcast while splashing around.

When I do settle into the rhythm of swimming, it relaxes and calms the emotions. The feel of water slipping over the body becomes almost hypnotic. And the change up among muscle groups brings a focus to the back and core abdomen areas. If you want "six pack abs" get in the pool and swim on frequent occasions. It's is a natural ongoing motion that tunes and refines your look.

*Stretching*

Before we end our conversation about fitness, I want to share something I have learned in the last year or so. As we go through a lifetime of diet and fitness goals, we need to become complete human beings.

For decades, my social identity was driven by my legs. Running and cycling ruled my life and my legs took the beating. Much of the rest of me suffered. I was delinquent in managing my assets in the best way possible. It took a while to get my schema repositioned, but now when I overview my objectives, stretching as a fitness activity pops to the top of the list.

Stretching is a formidable opponent to aging. As we age, our range of motion is reduced and we lose some percentage of balance. These setbacks come on slow and may be imperceptible at first, but over time it's a noted disadvantage.

I used to have a cursory stretching routine at the end of runs, about a minute or two in duration. That's not what I am suggesting. I wasn't strong enough, or directed enough in my own mind, to build a stretching routine that could alter me for the better. But there were others who were there to help. They came in the form of yoga instructors.

What was most important for me in a group yoga setting was that I was accepted. I attend sessions five days a week in a university recreation center. It's sometime hard to be seen as the one specimen in the room who can't twist into the pretzel formation sometimes called a "pose." But what I found is similar to my other athletic endeavors; stay calm and embrace limitations, while taking away the benefits that yoga provides.

There are several specific types of yoga. Some may be aggressive in nature, set in a hot environment, or incorporating couples sessions. When you research a possible yoga opportunity, run a search for "sun salutation." This is an easy progression of moves that we transition through several times in our morning yoga class. Yoga demands relaxation, a deep breathing pattern in relationship to poses, and sustained stretches that isolate specific areas of the body.

I have improved within my yoga practice. "Downward dog" is one of the most well-known yoga poses. I learned to keep a flat back and if that means keeping a bend in my legs, it's OK. I also bring yoga into my weight workouts using adapted warrior poses, incorporating a weight bar to challenge stability.

Another take away from yoga is that the return on investment (ROI) is subtle. It's not a high calorie burn activity, but as you practice over time, the body transforms. What I notice most is how I carry my body. Within daily moves, such as climbing stairs, getting up out of a couch, or swinging my leg over a bicycle, the balance and strength is improved. It's a lightness of being that brings confidence.

*Chapter summary*

- The pursuit of fitness endeavors can be all consuming and results oriented. Fitness can supplement your social identity, but it should not become your social identity.

- Develop your schema to assure that you are more that your sport. Weigh the investment needed against responsibility to career, family and other loved ones.

- The best fitness plan ever devised is the one you create and is sustainable over a long period of time.

- "Healthy, fit or light, pick two." It's almost impossible to attain all aspects of fitness at one time. Be gentle and gracious with yourself and the challenges ahead.

- Be aware of the modern fitness craze, but don't adhere to it. Research and develop your own vision for your Mind over Diet fitness program

- Embrace your abilities and place in the world, in each moment as they occur. Rest secure in your own identity, not the performances of others.

- There is no shortcut, fast results workout plans. Mind over Diet requires time and diligence.

- Understand the relationship between calories expended and various forms of exercise.

- Each form of exercise has a purpose but if the intensity is too high it may be unpleasant and produce a negative schema effect.

- Days off are an opportunity for breakdown in schema development.

- Self -negotiate and determine a minimum time for your workout session each day; then make sure you implement some form of exercise in that allocated time limit.

- Research and build your menu of exercise. Consider strength training, heart rate zones, running, bicycling, swimming and stretching. Understand the calories expended in each form of exercise. Develop a blend of activities for your Mind over Diet protocol.

# CHAPTER 7
## Digital food

You may have noted that a central theme in this book is "feed the mind, feed the body." Based on the input we choose, we can affect positive outcomes in our lives. A big piece that I can't recommend enough is a constant rebooting of the mind through digital audio messaging.

So, what are you listening to? What's loaded on your personal listening device? Common for many is a long playlist of songs. We prioritize, shuffle and repeat our favorite music. But as you become successful in your Mind over Diet quest and want to continually engage a sustainable path, there is a new frontier of content that will take you on a unique journey every day.

In an earlier chapter, I mentioned the act of associating, or disassociating, while performing endurance sport exercise. I may disassociate from my running, strength training or mountain biking experience. Rather, I'll opt to dig deeper into schema building by listening to a wide array of digital content.

I'm speaking about podcasts available on the Internet and digital audio books available through your local library. I have access to an immense database of knowledge. Dozens of new listening opportunities become available each day. And it's all free.

Most all of us are under time pressures. We try to pack 20 pounds of potatoes into a 10 pound bag each and every day. There's the need to work, to support our families, to invest in our personal well-being and now, to consistently move forward in building our schema and embracing social identities. There are opportunities to use the Internet and search favorite topics, but that takes an additional investment of time, which may not exist.

Consider setting the music aside and instead build your personal arsenal of mind enhancing digital content. There are no rules, no specific podcasters you must follow. I keep a list of about 20 podcasts on my daily sync list. When I plug in my listening device to charge, it updates all my choices. I head out into the day – and into my next workout – with fresh listening segments.

My choices are eclectic. I opt for podcasts that highlight ultrarunning, cycling, fitness lifestyles, comedy, politics, motorsport, religious and counter-religious topics. Many of my options and suggestions in this book have come from an enriched schema developed through exposure to these podcasts.

Listening to podcasts galvanizes my opinion of the fitness industry and motivates the Mind over Diet approach to my life. In many cases, the podcaster is adamant that her or his way is the only way. The message paints anyone with an alternative opinion as a buffoon.

I am a true believer in public debate. We can feed our minds with alternative points of view and then choose the good and bad in each argument. What I find healthy in this process is that you don't have to agree with each and every podcaster. Rather, it's the process of becoming better informed, testing ideas, and then making your own choices in your Mind over Diet journey.

Another guilty pleasure is audiobooks. I enjoy autobiographies written by famous rock music stars. I can recall one specific 50k race, on loops around a picturesque lake. My memories of that race are interlaced with a saucy rendition of the rock and roll lifestyle.

On another occasion, I was on a long woods touring session (that's what I call mountain biking, since I ride at a relaxed, safe pace) and was listening to a first person account from a famous British musician.

If you aren't currently a digital listener, there are several steps you can take to access this vast amount of material. Some brands of audio devices link to their own downloading library, while with others you can manually load the various podcasts as files. Check with your local library about their audiobook selections. Most offer accompanying software that can link your device to the library's loan system.

If you're searching online and spot a podcast you'd like to connect to, attempt to find the "RSS" feed for that podcast. The RSS feed is a specific Internet link that allows your device to read the incoming feeds for that show.

As with all things Mind over Diet, I'm not planning to direct you to my personal choices. If you do wish to read a bit more about comments I have made on podcasts, run a search within my personal blog mastercompetitor.blogspot.com.

If you choose to go digital while training, be safe. Keep the volume low so you are aware of everything around you. Also beware that due to insurance restrictions, some endurance sport events do not allow personal listening devices. Check ahead of time and respect the rules of the event promoter.

A positive association in my schema is a link between workouts and podcast listening. On some days I may not truly feel the push needed to get out the door, but seeing my listening device on the table is the first step in gearing up for the run, bike or gym. There are arguments to be made, stories to be told and news to be digested. All of that is one in the same with my exercise experience. Consider the opportunities and build your own personal digital portal.

*Chapter summary*

- If you choose to use a personal listening device, you have a choice regarding the content you absorb.
- Podcasts and audiobooks are plentiful and are free via the Internet.
- Your personal audio listening library will consistently reboot your schema.
- Podcasts present polarized points of view and create the debate necessary for an educated Mind over Diet process.
- Audiobooks can carry us into a pleasurable listening dimension on topics you enjoy.
- You can create a positive association between audio listening and daily exercise sessions.

# CHAPTER 8

## Afterthoughts

It's rather hard to believe we're at the end of this journey. I have been thinking about this book for several years and actually writing the manuscript over the past several months through countless edits and rewrites. I wish this book was "finished" but it is not. In Mind over Diet the information and subsequent knowledge never stops.

For example, I just came upon a U.S. government supported project that suggests a completely different calorie-burn approximation for weight loss. I also noted a new study that tells us excessive meat protein consumption is as dangerous as a pack-a-day smoking habit (this study also suggests .8 gram of protein per kilogram of body weight; I don't know how this compares to your personal analysis. I ran the math and my plant protein consumption is much higher that what this report recommends).

I haven't yet vetted this new material but it will surely raise the conversation level. It's up to each of us to determine what has salience in our lives. Bring the debate alive; don't allow others to interpret or make those decisions for you. Refresh your schema and draw conclusions that are authentic to your personal Mind over Diet plan.

Scientific reporting and research raises another issue. I considered writing an academic diet and fitness book, one that cited hundreds of experts from a variety of resources. But in its final version, Mind over Diet will only acknowledge one giant in the diet and fitness industry and that giant is you.

Every Mind over Diet advocate who takes the journey, who digs deep enough to build a proportional protein/carb/fat food plan, deserves to be respected in their accomplishment. And each individual who complements their diet plan with a daily fitness routine is credentialed as their own personal fitness trainer.

I often tell my students, "It's not what we know it's why we believe it." We are each an experiment of one and we are each validated in our personal scrutinizing process. Remember that it's left foot, right foot, left foot, right foot, striding methodically forward each day as we engage, tweak and adapt Mind over Diet to adapt to the situation. The journey isn't quick and the results aren't immediate. Mind over Diet has not been a short cut or fix-it plan. Rather, it's a set of tools that you can use to optimize your life.

I want to be transparent and disclose that recently, a dark cloud has hovered overhead. I have struggled in recent weeks, maybe due to stress, or possibly the unpredictable nature of the world around us, or maybe it's the simple process of aging.

These converged factors have muddied my calibrated eating plan. I fell into an illicit love affair with peanuts and powdered hot chocolate. My schema brought old files to the front; I began to equate food with comfort. A long, hard winter has forced months of indoor training and that has wreaked havoc with my social identity as an endurance athlete.

My conclusion is that my winter fitness plan – elliptical trainer, weight resistance and yoga – is necessary as part of an annual recovery plan. But my motivation exists through the running and cycling miles I engage the other eight months of the year. So it has started again, I'm back to my 10 mile per day runs. Going from zero to 60-70 miles a week has initially made me tired and beat up, but alive in spirit and hope. I find the social identity of running a motivating dimension. Small changes occur; the leanness comes back into my face and the drive to achieve seeps back into my inner being. There's a 50K warm up then another 100 mile run on the near horizon. I want to be open and receptive to the experience.

I'm also shaking up the food plan. I've been on protein bars and fruit for months. Small things bring big outcomes, so I'm ordering a really interesting salad container that will allow me to transport a raw salad and olive oil based lunch each day. I'm not sure that will be my direction forever, but the excitement of retesting and rebooting my system is never a bad decision. When we embrace the Mind over Diet model, we revise, change and alter our intake and activities to continue stepping forward.

Most all of us have been through many alternative seasons of life. Some hold great memories while others are painful to recall. What is real and true is that our schemas drive the order of our lives. Don't point fingers or blame the world around you. Rather, re-engaging in self-study and push new knowledge into your brain. Reorder the files in your schema to alter priorities. The dark clouds will part and sunshine will once again illuminate the paths you are walking.

When you hit the tough spots, lean hard into the Mind over Diet process and bring renewed energy into your life. You are a complex being that orders and processes dozens of variables. It's up to you regarding when and how those variables can be increased, decreased, or deleted. Feed the mind, feed the body and feel free to add new variables when research leads you to a fresh outlook.

I'd like to close with a saying that I try to engage on a daily basis:

"Not better or worse, just different."

Whether it's Paleo or vegan or fruitarian or weights or yoga or aerobic sport, proponents for each "club" have an assertive opinion. They will usually declare their program as the best or only alternative. We can listen to, and respect each argument and then weigh the essence. Let's create our own hybrid models. We don't have to rank-file and choose winners; rather, we can blend and moderate and rest in our own conclusions.

The Mind over Diet journey is bigger than diet and fitness; there are other opportunities waiting. Think of the many polarized factions in society. We have screaming heads on TV cable channels and no one seems to get along. We have lost our appetite for civil, social debate. And if there's a lesson in all of this, it is harbored in the fact that many opinions exist and in most cases, they are not better or worse, just different. Let's all become the voice of reason, setting an example for others. We can teach those around us to sift information carefully and present interpretations from both points of view.

Care about others. Demonstrate the intensity of your effort, how you came to develop your daily food plan and why your fitness sessions make sense for you. When we inspire others to embrace an active sport lifestyle, our passion will continue to burn strong.

Above all, have fun. Enjoy your exercise and fitness activities every day. Mix it up, try strength training on one day and mix yoga the next. Reach high and renew the Mind over Diet experience. It's an ongoing form of joy and reward.

When the "new you" emerges from Mind over Diet, friends and acquaintances will ask, "What happened?" When that moment comes, stop, take a deep breath, and enjoy the world around you. Then smile and inquire, "Have you ever taken the naked test?"

# CHAPTER 9

## About the author

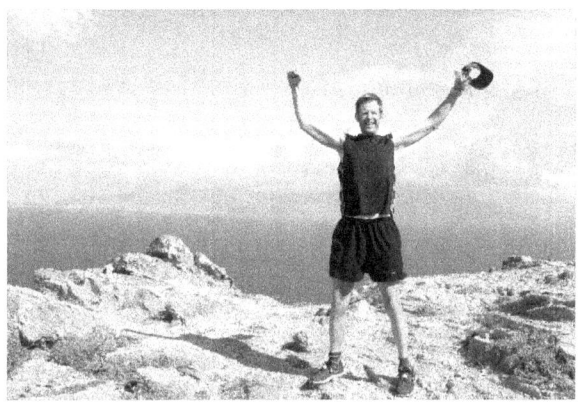

Thomas Mueller was a self-described bench-warmer in all forms of sport. He was afraid of gym class in grade school (might fall off the trampoline), was cut from the B squad in high school basketball, then went out for and was subsequently cut from the hockey team in university. There was no sport in which Mueller excelled – until he stumbled into the world of endurance sport.

Mueller was overweight, sluggish, and consuming too much alcohol as part of his public relations lifestyle. He craved change and in the fall of 1983, purchased an inexpensive bicycle and began to ride and sporadically run. What started as a waddle soon turned to a jog and Mueller was motivated to enhance the experience. He began adhering to a low calorie diet and in the fall of 1983, transitioned from 213 pounds to his eventual weight of 165.

Identifying with cycling and running created an edifying experience Mueller had never known. The days of sitting on the bench and being identified as an inappropriate performer were over. In endurance sport, each day is an event and everyone who participates is the winner.

Mueller entered his first race in 1984 and completed the 10 mile run and 30 mile bike segments. In the years following, Mueller found a deep passion for short course triathlon racing, marathon running, ultradistance running, road cycling and mountain biking. In the past 30 years, Mueller has completed over 150 endurance sport events. Some of his key accomplishments include six (6) finishes at the Mohican 100-mile run in Ohio, eight (8) finishes at the Ice Age 50-mile in Wisconsin, approximately seventy-five (75) marathon finishes (including New York, Chicago and the Marine Corps in D.C.) and two (2) completed *Great Bicycle Ride Across Wisconsin* tours.

Mueller has been a Brooks Sports ambassador for over 20 years. He adheres to the "Inspire Daily" brand identity and promotes his active running and fitness lifestyle through local bike and running clubs.

On a professional and academic front, Mueller built an extensive career in business development through event and affinity marketing. He holds a journalism degree from the University of Wisconsin, a MBA from Otterbein University, and a PhD in Communication from the University of Florida.

Mueller's international experience began in the early 1980's as a writer and photographer for Cycle News East, where he covered motorcycle sporting events in the United States and Europe. Later, as part of his MBA study, Mueller participated in an international economics study in Helsinki, Finland and St. Petersburg, Russia. It was during this trip that Mueller drafted a topical paper on free-market Russia and the opportunities that have emerged since the country formed independent republics in 1991.

He returned to Russia on an academic and business speaking tour the following year and traveled in the southwestern region of the country near Rostov-on Don. The tour interacted with students and business leaders in several communities. More recently, Mueller has participated in several University of Florida international study abroad programs.

Mueller opened a public relations agency and served the Wrangler Brand in Greensboro, NC. He was responsible for Wrangler's promotional work in NASCAR with Dale Earnhardt, professional rodeo, and stadium Supercross motorcycle racing. He later opened Sport Management, Inc. and went on to sell and manage over $5 million in corporate sponsorships.

Mueller was a marketing director at Mercury Marine and then became Director of Professional Competition for the American Motorcyclist Association. He earned an accredited sporting steward's license with the International Motorcycling Federation and went on assignment for FIM business in South America and Europe.

Mueller was also employed by Wasserman Media Group, a Los Angeles - based entertainment company. He was an account supervisor and was responsible for integrating Rally America auto sport racing into the ESPN X Games.

Mueller completed his PhD in 2009 and that same year assumed his current role as assistant professor in communication at Appalachian State University in Boone, North Carolina. He teaches a variety of courses in advertising, media planning, research, and the social effects of media.

His research focuses on the psychological dimensions and related motivators among endurance sport, motorsport, corporate social responsibility and the university student loan process, among others.

**Want more?**

If you'd like to explore more opportunities with the Mind over Diet life process, watch for updates on mastercompetitor.blogspot.com or mindoverdiet.blogspot.com.

Also learn more about Dr. Mueller at profwriter.com.

Dr. Mueller is available for:

- Public and corporate speaking events
- Sponsorship development and analysis
- Sport and entertainment event consultation
- Fitness event guide and mentor
- Corporate wellness initiatives
- Group fitness analysis and planning
- Consumer research
- E-Learning program development